The **FIR**

Fight Insulin Resistance with Strength Training

Or

Your Optimal Exercise Guide to

Diabetes
Prediabetes
Metabolic Syndrome,
Cholesterol,
and Cardiovascular Disease

A Science based Approach

William Y. Shang, M.D.

To Len and Eden,

Best wishes.

Dr. Shang

Shang Publishing
Library of Congress Control Number: 2016909695

- ## Medical Disclaimer:

All content found within including text, images, software, other formats are
for informational purposes only. The content is not intended to be a
substitute for professional medical advice, diagnosis, or treatment. Always
seek the advice of your physician or other qualified health provider, trainer,
physical therapist with any questions you may have regarding a medical
condition. Never disregard professional medical advice or delay in seeking it
because of something you have read in this book. It is always advisable to
seek qualified advice before embarking upon a new exercise regimen,
especially if you have known medical issues.

If you think you may have a medical emergency, call your doctor, go to the
emergency department immediately. The author is not your personal
physician nor sufficiently familiar with your health situation to decide
whether the specific exercises are appropriate for any particular person. The
author is not able to specifically recommend or endorse any specific tests,
physicians, exercise, opinions, or other information that may suitable in your
own case. Reliance on any information provided is solely at your own risk.

Links to educational content not created by the author are to be taken at
your own risk.

Table of Contents:

Preface

This book is written for the motivated person who would like to take control or be active participants in their health. Some of patients upon hearing of their new diagnosis, eagerly ask their doctors what they can do – without having to take medications. I'm always heartened by this "take charge" attitude. However, too many physicians either underestimate what exercise is capable of accomplishing, or assume patients lack the will to change the trajectory of their lives.

If the physician initially takes out the prescription pad, the impetus for self-improvement through exercise fades almost to an afterthought. My aim is to intercede at this juncture, educate and inspire the reader to realize there is a possibility of beating the diagnosis rap of Metabolic Syndrome. The science presented in this book is sound and the exercise methods supported by the American Diabetes Association and the American College of Sports Medicine, among other professional medical organizations. Surprisingly however, even the primary thrust of the book may be entirely new ground for even the knowledgeable physicians.

Specifically targeted, tailored and dosed exercise as a treatment, not merely as disease prevention is foreign territory for most physicians, falling more into the field of exercise kinesiology. Experts in the field of exercise kinesiology, may not have detailed knowledge of cell pathophysiology however. Trainers exhort, teach and lead exercises better than others, but might only have a smattering grasp of internal medicine. Physicians have detailed understanding of drugs and surgery, but little beyond generalities when it comes to exercise. As an institutions of health and medicine, we are failing. We are attempting to treat an epidemic lifestyle-induced disease with pharmacology and dietary tweaking, when the primary cause is sedentary habits, overeating, and where strenuous adversity has been nearly engineered out of existence. Sure, walking and increased activity are today's buzzwords of healthcare providers. But, why aren't the best exercise practices from successful research studies common knowledge and routine practice?

Our healthcare system is a pharmaceutical and procedure driven industry offering consumable diets, supplements, drugs and surgery. Our entertainment-consumer driven economy emphasizes profit, promotion of quick results while promising minimal effort, sprinkled with fun. Consequently, little monetary incentive exists within this framework to research a low-cost method of treating a lifestyle-induced disease. Therefore, as a society, we find ourselves with the deck stacked against exercise as a first-line emphasized, and funded treatment. Luckily, countries outside of the US have taken up the cause of advancing exercise science.

Hence, I felt compelled to write this book. During the course of researching and composing, I would regularly feel egged onward. One instance was an incomplete and misleading a *New York Times* article my sister forwarded, about the winners of *The Biggest Loser*. In the popular television show, contestants compete to see who can lose the most weight over the shortest time. Sadly, many of the biggest losers on this show became the "great big" gainers after the cameras departed. This article offered no explanation other than the usual mystical homilies and seemed to refute the First Law of Thermodynamics. (The First Law of Thermodynamics otherwise known as the Law of Conservation of Energy, states that energy cannot be created or destroyed in an isolated system.) I feel frustrated by these medically inaccurate articles – another missed opportunity to educate the public. Researchers *know* the reasons for weight re-gain and why weight loss is difficult, yet a majority of medical professionals do not. As an example, most healthcare professionals incorrectly answer the questions, "Why does the basal metabolic rate decrease with a low-calorie diet and aerobic exercise weight loss?" and "Obese patients have high insulin levels, how could that affect your treatment of weight loss?"

Later that same day after receiving my sister's email, I worked out at a crowded Planet Fitness, *The Biggest Loser's* major sponsor on their busiest day – "Pizza Day," when they give out free pizza to all members. Whatever the motivation for TV contestants to compete, viewers to watch or gym members to show up, motivation appears misdirected. The reasons and optimal methods for dealing with the greatest healthcare crisis mankind faces – insulin resistance, remains bizarrely obscure and sub-optimally treated by most people attempting exercise. I will provide answers, not my opinion, translating basic science and research paper findings.

Along the way, I wish to share insights into what is normal aging. We have lost accurate points of reference with aging. Outward manifestations of insulin resistance such as, ebbing strength, deteriorating mental faculties, rising rates of cancer, diabetes, atherosclerosis, and high blood pressure, are so common that we've practically mistaken them for normality. Our sedentary, assistive technological lifestyle has conspired with the sanitized phrase "risk factor" to confuse our understanding. Finally, we have a misplaced faith in labs and imaging to confidently assert what is health and what is fitness.

You cannot see that yellow plaque on your aorta dissolving. You cannot see the Type II muscle fiber increasing in size in your thigh. You cannot see nerves reconnecting to muscle cells. You cannot see the GLUT-4 glucose transporter molecule packets fusing with the muscle cell membrane, reversing the effects of insulin resistance. As an expert with the microscope, I will share with you the wonders of your body and how regain what is rightfully your evolutionary heritage.

So while scientifically validated but less publicized, this exercise prescription still requires a commitment to continuous self-improvement – the key ingredient **only you** can bring to the mix. The lure of free pizza to make the trip to the gym is not a sustainable reason. Motivation   is easier to sustain with a firm understanding of pathology or how things go wrong. The discussion would not be complete without following up with an exercise plan, which is later in the book – an exercise regimen designed to address the pathology. If you could see the microscopic and internal body pathologic changes that result from Metabolic Syndrome, you would not falter nor hesitate to exercise. I would like to believe that you are among those who will strive to care for your body after gaining a firm understanding of the why's and how's.

If you would like to take a shortcut, read the Executive Summary. Skip to the back, and start the exercise regimen. In time, come back and read your way forward as the spirit moves you. Meanwhile, imagine all those hormones, cells and chemical processes all getting back to alignment with each rep.

Chapter 1: Executive Summary

Even a simplified science book may be difficult to plow through. Medical theories can be difficult to follow, especially without a biology background. If you read this Executive Summary, you will have covered the key points. Since concepts are often captured by specific vocabulary and medical words can be challenging, consider looking through the glossary first, to smooth your reading.

Doctors often recommend diet and exercise to treat prediabetes, diabetes, Metabolic Syndrome and worsening cholesterol. And while many diet books exist, only a few are guides to exercise and are rarely backed by research. This book seeks to fill this gap and dispel the notion that atherosclerosis, slowing metabolism, elevated lipids, rising glucose and decreasing strength are unavoidable consequences of aging. Time does "take a toll," but not nearly to the extent you might have been led to believe. You have the power to change the course of your body's metabolism by following the exercise regimen in this book. Even if you are not overweight, but not doing resistance exercise, it's probable you can markedly improve your metabolism in all the above risk categories.

A few years ago, leading medical organizations established a point system for cardiovascular risk factors. When this risk scale applied to the US population, roughly 60% of the population over the age of 50, have the blandly named, Metabolic Syndrome. "Metabolic Syndrome," is an epidemic. Those who have it are silently developing atherosclerosis or damage to the heart and blood vessels which reveal themselves as strokes, heart attacks, high blood pressure and dementia. In most cases, the insidious, ongoing organ and blood vessel damage cannot be discovered through testing as it is microscopic and cannot be seen even with modern technology. As someone who performed autopsies on accident victims, I can vouch that damage is taking place. In this way, the term, "risk factor," is misleading because the catastrophic event has not occurred, but the seeds for the event have sprouted.

Physicians know elevated blood pressure represents a continuum of risk starting below the traditionally advertised 140/90 mmHg. Many believe insulin resistance of blood vessel cells causes high blood pressure. The same continuum of insulin resistance damage holds true for the diagnostic fasting blood sugar threshold of 100mg/dL for diabetes. Caucasians with a BMI of >25, and Asians of >23 should be screened for prediabetes. Excess visceral central fat, (fat which is around internal organs) which appears as a pear-shaped body contour is believed to cause insulin resistance. An abnormal blood cholesterol panel and triglyceride are additional criteria for Metabolic Syndrome. One or more of these risk factors increase the possibility of silent atherosclerotic blood vessel disease, increased risk of cancer, heart attack, stroke and dementia.

Many people are in treatment limbo when it comes to Metabolic Syndrome. In the early stages, the adverse medication side effects outweigh the immediate disease risk. Therefore physicians may be hesitant to treat until a later stage. Prediabetes is not an early stage of disease, but mid-stage, occurring only after the pancreas has peaked insulin production and not kept pace with an upwardly spiraling insulin resistance. After a few more years, insulin producing pancreatic Beta cells will begin to die of exhaustion. Each passing year with diabetes closes the window of opportunity to lessen the load on the pancreas and return the body to a normal metabolism. An earlier commitment to lifelong exercise increases the chances of reversing damage and the underlying insulin resistance.

Are these diseases or just part of normal aging? Understanding this requires us to frame the questions properly. Some are under the misconception that diabetes is two diseases, or conceived as simply pancreatic, or as a sugar dietary disorder. Medical providers might misconceive drugs as treating the underlying disorder rather than an intermediary or surrogate.

Because of the limitations of a 15-minute visit, many physicians have almost given up encouraging life-altering, lifestyle change and exercise. To quote the American College of Sports Medicine, "Exercise is Medicine." Exercise when tailored like a prescription, can cure or ameliorate damage which has been wrongly attributed to aging.

The optimal exercise regimen is resistance exercise added to the more commonly known aerobic exercise component. The two forms of exercise have mutually complementary effects on muscle. The principal abnormality in Metabolic Syndrome and its follow-on Type 2 diabetes is insulin resistance, not high glucose or LDL. Insulin resistance is not tested as part of a regular exam testing. Many patients and healthcare professionals do not conceptualize this as the primary underlying and correctable problem. Aging has been wrongly blamed for much of the glucose and lipid toxicity glucolipotoxicity of insulin resistance. Metabolic Syndrome and the body's resistance to insulin result from lifestyle deviations from our evolutionary heritage. Sedentary behavior and the absence of a vigorous muscular exercise has led to a metabolic derangement for most people. By the time glucose rises above 100mg/dL, insulin has peaked and the pancreas is exhausted. About an eight year window exists when a concerted effort can save the pancreas and prevent the disease from continuing on a downward course.

The amount of skeletal muscle declines with age. Skeletal muscle performs a valuable and under-recognized role in metabolism. Without regular vigorous challenges, muscles become a dysfunctional metabolic organ contributing to insulin resistance. Resistance training can reverse muscle's insulin resistance, restoring normal metabolism at any age and to an astonishing degree. Recent research has found exercising large core muscle groups to exhaustion as key to reversing insulin resistance.

Obesity is not a requirement for insulin resistance. About 16% of severely insulin resistance individuals are not overweight. Sarcopenia induced insulin resistance may explain the many who have heart attacks without have no identifiable risk factors. One rule of thumb, if the triglyceride to HDL ratio is >3.0 for men, then it is likely insulin has been working overtime just to keep glucose levels down. Keeping track of your historical triglyceride level may give you a gauge of insulin resistance, especially if triglycerides have been increasing.

For those starting out with a BMI above 32, aerobic exercise may be a good start. Before too long, a weight loss plateau often stymies further progress. Weight loss without preservation of skeletal muscle mass usually leads to regaining that initial weight loss. Basal metabolic rates are mostly determined by skeletal muscle mass and the energy required to make new muscle fibers can be substantially increased with resistance exercise. Without incorporation of resistance exercise into a regular exercise routine, daily caloric needs generally decline with loss of muscle mass. This scenario is all too familiar for those who attempt diet, or diet plus aerobic exercise for weight loss. The resulting yo-yo weight changes enter into a negative feedback loop where every cycle makes weight loss more difficult.

Progressive resistance training likely requires more than the present RDA dietary protein recommendations of 0.8 grams/kg of body weight per day. Muscles of those older than 60 are less responsive to dietary protein compared with younger muscle, a phenomenon termed Anabolic Resistance. For older exercisers seeking to increase skeletal muscle mass, increasing daily total protein to 1.2-1.4 gm/ kg of body weight per day should be of benefit. Seniors often can benefit from a high-quality, whey protein rich supplement.

A proper exercise regimen is far superior to physical activity because it is prescriptive. Like a scientifically based structure medical treatment plan, the goal is to effect permanent adaptations within the body. Some highly motivated individuals who can routinely perform an exercise regimen to achieve the stated objectives. Studies have shown that the majority of people will require trainers for education on proper technique, provide incentive, encouragement, as well as prevent injury. Injury is a common reason for discontinuation and is usually related to poor form, advancing too rapidly for joints, ligaments and soft tissue to keep pace with a faster-growing muscle. Nonetheless, numerous studies have shown properly performed aerobic and resistance exercise as part of a structured regimen, can decrease waistlines, improve cholesterol numbers, glucose and blood pressure and reverse insulin resistance.

Chapter 2: My own journey

Why this book?

Why this book? The short answer: because I, the doctor personally needed to find answers.

Several years ago, I found myself with a fasting blood sugar slowly drifting upward. An fasting blood sugar greater than 100mg/dL is one of the criteria for prediabetes and Metabolic Syndrome. My glucose level had been fine throughout my thirties, but toward the last part of my forties, it had gone into the 90mg/dL range and by my fifties, often into the low 100mg/dL range. As a physician, I had always been conscious of my own health. I'm an avid cyclist and on cold rainy New York days, work out at home on an elliptical or go to the local Y to swim. Although my grandmother was diagnosed with diabetes late in her years, I wasn't aware of a strong family history for diabetes

Even more curiously, I have never been overweight. My weight has been pretty much the same throughout college, medical school, Air Force, general practice years, pathology residency and private practice as a community hospital pathologist and county coroner physician, up until Cornell University. To make matters worse, along with my rising glucose, my triglycerides were rising. Elevated triglycerides, a fat blood test is another flag, warning sign and criteria for Metabolic Syndrome. Somehow, I was on the cusp of joining the ranks of my patients with prediabetes, part of Metabolic Syndrome.

If you are like me, we're in good company. In fact, we are probably part of a dubious majority. After age 65, about half of us have a fasting glucose level greater than 100mg/dL, meeting one of the criteria for Metabolic Syndrome. Here is the criteria for Metabolic Syndrome in chart form:

Criteria for Metabolic Syndrome

3 or more of the following:

1. Waist circumference >40" in men and > 34.5" in women (Asians males >35," Asian females >33.5")
2. Triglycerides ≥150 mg/dl or using drugs for treatment
3. HDL <40 mg/dl in men and < 50 mg/dl in women or under treatment
4. Systolic blood pressure >130 mmHg or diastolic blood pressure ≥85 mmHg or under treatment
5. Fasting Glucose ≥100 mg/dl or under treatment for diabetes

(2005 Grundy, ATPIII Revised Criteria)

The criteria for Metabolic Syndrome is met when at least three of five of the following medical conditions are present: abdominal (central) obesity, high serum triglycerides, elevated blood pressure, elevated fasting plasma glucose, and subnormal high-density lipoprotein (HDL) levels. About a third of all adult age Americans have Metabolic Syndrome and nearly 60% fulfill the criteria by age 50. Metabolic Syndrome thereby fits the very definition of the word *epidemic,* as the prevalence of Metabolic Syndrome has been rapidly increasing each decade. If this were an infectious disease, the CDC (Center for Disease Control) would have a serious problem quarantining all of us!

"The Deadly Quartet" or Why should you care?

In 1989, Dr. Norman Kaplan coined the term "Deadly Quartet" to define and bring to public attention the known and *modifiable* risk factors for cardiovascular disease, the number one killer. Cardiovascular disease encompasses diseases of the blood vessels and heart, such as narrowing of the blood vessels, atherosclerosis and blockage. We commonly recognize cardiovascular disease as heart attacks, strokes and thrombophlebitis to name the most common bad actors.

Early in the 1990's on the term SYNDROME X was tried, but probably didn't stick for plain weirdness. The term *Metabolic Syndrome* seems to be here for good. *Metabolic Syndrome* identifies modifiable risk factors for heart attack, stroke and blood vessel atherosclerosis. *Modifiable* means factors quite possibly within our control. A "syndrome" is a group of symptoms that consistently occur together. The "S" in AIDS, for instance, stands for the constellations of "symptoms" before Human Immunodeficiency Virus (HIV) was discovered. We knew certain diseases tended to present in the same patient together. *Metabolic Syndrome* identifies the clustering of obesity, high blood pressure, prediabetes, diabetes, elevated blood lipids, heart attack, stroke, dementia, fatty liver and cancers such as breast and colon in the same patients.

While I don't like the term *Metabolic Syndrome* for its

nondescript sounding name, it's a useful term because it tells you that the disease complex primarily involves metabolism. If given a chance to rename the disease complex, I'd prefer INSULIN RESISTANCE SYNDROME – because the common thread among the diseases appears to be insulin resistance. Insulin is part of the body's energy management system and therefore affects every cell in the body. The seemingly unconnected collection of diseases caused by resistance to insulin, therefore, shouldn't be surprising. Insulin-resistance is not synonymous with Metabolic Syndrome. <u>The three criteria of Metabolic Syndrome only become fulfilled after a moderately high degree of insulin-resistance.</u> We'll talk later about what is and causes insulin resistance. Suffice now to say, when a constellation of diseases become commonplace, we often mistake them as normal – in this case aging. Insulin resistance is the hidden culprits or abettors behind what we thought were diseases of aging.

The notion coronary atherosclerosis (atherosclerosis occurring with the arteries of the heart) was abnormal aging did not occur to me until I learned an interesting fact during a casual conversation with the animal pathologists at Cornell's veterinary school. According to them, only birds might develop narrowing of the heart blood vessels. Carnivores and obligate carnivores, animals who only eat meat, do not have heart attacks. Humans, on the other hand, are now eating and living in a fashion, unlike any other period since we as a species walked out of Africa and colonized the earth. Mankind's DNA has wide genetic diversity, sometimes resulting in rare, bizarre diseases. In our shared history, epidemics are caused by infections.

Any widespread disease such as Type 2 diabetes is not primarily a genetic problem but a maladaptation, a deviation from our historic lifestyle. Most books and media have focused on dietary changes but the evidence more strongly indicates an activity maladaptation. Prior to the last century, isolated tribes survived and prospered on a limited variety of food. Eskimos eat an extremely high-fat, green-leafy-vegetable-poor diet, for example. I suggest considering *Metabolic Syndrome* to be a predominantly an activity maladaptation, in other words, our bodies are not adapting well to the low exertional levels of modern life.

While proper diet is important, please consider the consumer market industries which tend to overemphasize the relative importance of eating. Please recall in the 1960's, the sugar industry paid scientists to play down links between sugar and heart disease and promote fat as the culprit, derailing dietary recommendations for five decades. (Kearns 2016)

According to the 2014 World Health Organization, (WHO) *Global status report on noncommunicable diseases,* we have transitioned as a species. Noninfectious diseases now cause more diseases than communicable, maternal, perinatal and nutritional conditions combined. Interpreted from another angle, vaccines, clean water, antibiotics have lifted us out of the jungle. The largest epidemic in world or US history doesn't comes from a virus or bacteria. Atherosclerotic related death from heart disease and stroke are more than twice that of cancer. We are our own worst enemy. The WHO report further claims that the "metabolic risk factor globally is elevated blood pressure . . . followed by overweight and obesity and raised blood glucose." When diseases are part of an evolving syndrome, there is a tendency for one to appear first with others evolving only to declare themselves later. If one or more of the Metabolic Syndrome's *dummy lights,* or if you prefer *idiot lights* on the dashboard are flashing, the time to change the your body's maintenance schedule is now. Please don't wait for the car to end up in a ditch.

When lab reports qualified me for two but not three of the *Metabolic Syndrome* criteria, I became concerned. Don't be fooled by semantics. Risk factors and *Metabolic Syndrome* don't translate into "nothing is happening yet," most likely it means "something's bad in the works." As someone who has performed autopsies on car accident victims, lives tragically cut short, I saw atherosclerosis long before it could appear on imaging tests.

Let's look at the case against insulin resistance as the cause of atherosclerosis. When studies attempting to "normalize" glucose levels in diabetes did not reduce the number of heart attacks and strokes, researchers began to question insulin. Some diabetics became dangerously hypoglycemic as higher levels of insulin were used, while not gaining proportional lifespan or any decrease in complications. Some researchers began to wonder if the stage for blood vessel damage had been set in the prediabetic stage, an earlier phase of the same disease process as Type 2 diabetes. Is insulin resistance beginning in prediabetes phase damaging? Dr. Ausk followed over 5500 patients without diabetes or obesity, who had documented insulin resistance and found increased death rates at the twelve year mark. (Ausk 2010) Earlier Dr. Haffner compared prediabetics who were insulin resistant compared to those who had not developed insulin resistance. Haffner concluded factors causing atherosclerosis, "in the prediabetic state are mainly seen in insulin-resistant subjects." (Haffner 2000)

My car crash victims were not diagnosed with insulin-resistant atherosclerosis while alive, in part because insulin resistance is not a test a doctor typically orders, rather, it is a research study test. Insulin levels and resistance are not routinely tested. Sometimes a test known as C-peptide is used as a surrogate test for insulin, but almost never as a test for insulin resistance. Patients can be largely identified as insulin resistant if they meet some of the Metabolic Syndrome criteria. Most of the damage insulin resistance inflicts on the body is through blood vessel damage. Ongoing atherosclerotic damage is the common thread linking diabetes as the leading cause of kidney failure, poor circulation leading to amputations, and blindness according to the 2014 WHO report. Presently, high blood pressure, obesity, hyperglycemia and hyperlipidemia are thought to have the same common root – insulin resistance. Insulin resistance should be addressed through the primary cause – an abnormal lifestyle.

The traditional advice given to those with Metabolic Syndrome is to lose weight. More than four out of five people with diabetes are overweight. Well, that didn't make much sense in my case - I can still fit into my USAF flight suit from my twenties. The most common sense advice typically heard is to make changes in what passes between your lips: weight loss by restricting calories. While good advice, this is an example where theory and practice diverge. High insulin levels in obesity stymie most attempts at weight loss for reasons which will make sense when we talk about metabolism later.

Although I agree with the dietary recommendations of the American Diabetes Association (ADA), I like to be somewhat contrarian and say, "You are NOT, however, simply what you eat!" As a physician who started practicing in the 1980's, I was part of the mass misinformation campaign regarding dietary cholesterol. We were taught to tell patients that eating high cholesterol foods led to high blood cholesterol.

The cholesterol story of Dr. Ancel Keys and a previously obscure organization is a fascinating story worth briefly retelling. Dr. Keys was a prominent physiologist who was influential in creating the K-ration and Mediterranean Diet. In publishing the *Seven Countries Study* which appeared to show that dietary fat was correlated to heart attack death, he inexplicably withheld data from his entire set of twenty-two countries. The American Heart Association, which received monetary support from multiple companies including the pharmaceutical industry, supported the notion that a high fat diet would lead to coronary heart disease. This, in turn, led the US Government to recommend a low-fat diet in order to prevent heart disease. Only in 2015, did the US Government's Dietary Guidelines change "because available evidence shows no appreciable relationship between consumption of dietary cholesterol and serum cholesterol. . . . Cholesterol is not a nutrient of concern for overconsumption." As it turns out only a minority, maybe less than a quarter of patients can reduce serum cholesterol by decreasing fat intake. Nutritional studies, like the *Seven Countries Study,* are population-based studies and highly prone to mistaking cause for effect, even in the absence of deliberate bias, perhaps explaining why it seems as if the medical media reports that the same food is good one week, and toxic the next.

The science of biochemistry is a little more straightforward compared to nutrition. About 85% of the body's cholesterol is manufactured internally. As a general rule, the liver and the gut bacteria re-purpose nutritional needs, except for essential fats, amino acids and vitamins. In my own case, my diet consists of a nutrient dense, sensible diet. I wasn't running afoul of any of the diet recommendations - whether in fat content or the outmoded glycemic index of foods. So why was I sliding into this morass? The key to figuring out this puzzle is to go back to the Metabolic Syndrome criteria and ask, "Why is there a lower BMI <23 cutoff for Asians (East Indians, Southeast Asians and east Asians)?" and "Why does a non-obese person, the one out of five get diabetes? I will give you a clue now and the answer later. Asians have less muscle per pound than Caucasians. (Sattar 2015) Since I can write my own prescriptions, maybe I should prescribe myself medication?

Maybe you can just give me a pill?!

The metabolic system bears the marks of being cobbled

together by evolution. A disturbance in the system affects fuel conversion, distribution, parsing, and utilization. A single gene defect disease such as sickle cell anemia, might in theory be cured after some nifty DNA cutting and pasting. When the body's fuel system veers off track, defects cascade in a series of maladaptive runaway reactions. My first class of medical school pharmacology opened with the professor asking, "How do medications work? Magic?" Medications work because they substitute or interfere at some level of the body's mechanisms or physiology. Drugs work superbly for single cause problems, such as antibiotics directed at a specific bacterial cell wall. Not as clear is how a single drug for diabetes can halt the downstream effects of many moving parts gone awry. Does it make sense to initially treat a lifestyle-induced disease whose root problem is a deviation from human evolutionary heritage with medications – does that make sense?

Let's look at an example. Thiazolidinediones are a drug class designed to reverse the basic problem in Type 2 diabetes of resistance to insulin. Avandia (Rosiglitazone) and Actos (Pioglitazone) are commonly prescribed versions of these drugs. They act upon on PPAR receptors in the body and muscle, which happens to be also one of the known signaling pathways through which exercise reverses insulin resistance. The 2008 DREAM (Diabetes REduction Assessment with Ramipril and Rosiglitazone Medication) study found the risk of progressing to Type 2 diabetes within three years was reduced by 60%. (DREAM Team, 2008) Incidentally, this is nearly identical to 58% reduction with exercise in the Finnish

Diabetes Prevention Study and the Diabetes Prevention Program. (Tuomilehto 2001, Knowler 2002) Exercise performed as well as medication. Why not just take the medication? Rosiglitazone was found to have been associated with more heart failure. The patients don't care so much about progressing to diabetes compared to experiencing a heart failure, which the authors de-emphasized. Subsequent letters to the editor pointed out the glaring contradiction. While the reviewing FDA narrowly approved Rosiglitazone, Europe and India have banned Rosiglitazone's use. Please be aware drug companies fund studies as well as have representatives sit on government approval boards – scientific research abounds with bias.

Medications are not the same as exercise because they usually act upon a single moving part, may treat a lab value and have idiosyncratic as well as known side effects. In prediabetes, healthcare providers generally do not prescribe medications, although metformin sometimes is considered. Aside from metformin, I am not aware of medication a physician can offer to the non-obese person in this limbo, gray zone of prediabetes.

Presently, American Diabetes Association (ADA) guidelines suggest that patients with a BMI of at least 35 kg/m^2, who are younger than age 60, as well as some women with gestational diabetes might be reasonable candidates for metformin. Metformin mimics benefits of exercise because it acts upon one of exercise's metabolic reaction pathways. Initially, researchers from the University of Alberta found those patients taking metformin and exercising had different results from those simply exercising. Metformin appears to cap exercise performance because patients taking metformin reach the same heart rate or exercise intensity at lower exertion levels. (Boule 2011 & Boule 2013) In other words, early evidence suggests metformin might blunt some of the full benefits of exercise when improving insulin sensitivity and decreasing inflammation. To answer the question which is better, one head-to-head study published in the New England Journal concluded exercise bested metformin for preventing the transition from prediabetes to diabetes. (Knowler 2002) The study however, only utilized aerobic exercise. Since experts recommend aerobic plus resistance exercise, a future study will demonstrate an even greater superiority of exercise over metformin. Metformin has a dosage, which overtime generally increases as prediabetes progresses. By contrast, the physiologic improvements triggered by exercise progressively decreases the need for medication in prediabetes. Conceptually, this last point trumps all other considerations of price, or medication side effects. At this time, it is not entirely clear whether medications are helpful in prediabetes in all circumstances, although they may delay or lengthen the time to develop diabetes.

In my case, I decided to address the elevated triglycerides by putting myself on Niacin. Also known as Vitamin B3, this was available without a prescription. Niacin was approved by the FDA in 1997 for controlling lipids. A known side effect of Niacin is skin flushing, which helped me empathize more closely with women going through menopause. Liver damage is a more concerning side effect of Niacin, so regular blood tests are necessary. On the plus side, doctors knew Niacin raised HDL, (High Density Lipoprotein) the "good" fraction of cholesterol as well as lowered triglycerides. Studies have shown high HDL levels and low triglyceride levels are associated with have fewer heart attacks. Shockingly, multiyear medical studies following patients taking Niacin by 2011 didn't bear out the expected results. (Bodin 2011). Despite enduring uncomfortable flushing and regular blood tests, patients did not benefit from fewer heart attacks. The moral of the story: treating a lab value is not the same as treating a disease. A good or improving lab value does not in all cases, mean someone is healthy or healthier. For years, the medical community mistook a surrogate laboratory test result for health and made the mistake of thinking that fixing a lab value would fix a disease. Since the publication of this analysis, Niacin in all its forms has since been removed by order of the FDA.

Recurrent Pitfalls in the Medical World

A sort of "Undesired Situation" occurs when the medical community is unwittingly fooled by a coinciding lab value, analogous to Niacin. Far too often, correlation is mistaken for the underlying cause, causation. Please follow along with the diagram above. In this case, a test result such as HDL is known to correlate with heart disease. Niacin is known to raise HDL, however, higher levels of HDL aren't accompanied by fewer heart attacks. The drug has been acting upon HDL levels which are coincident to some upstream cause of heart attacks. As a result, doctors been treating patients without the desired result –

fooled!

The Undesired Situation: Fooled Again!

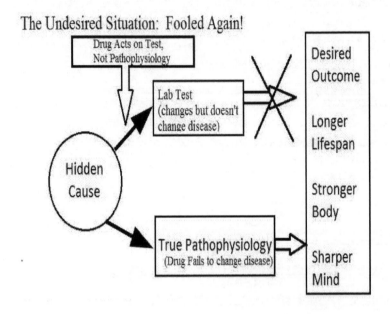

Compare this with the "Desired Situation." In this ideal circumstance, physicians accurately understand the

The Desired Situation: It all makes sense!

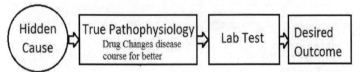

pathophysiology, which is the how physiology goes awry and disease evolves. Furthermore, a precise and accurate test can gauge the changes. Finally, we have a drug, treatment, or exercise which can improve the disease. By the way, Pathology is my specialty, the study of pathophysiology as well as Laboratory Medicine, the precise and accurate measurement of tests. The overall goal is to an accurate picture akin to the diagram labeled, "The Desired Situation: It all makes sense!"

The Niacin debacle tells us how easy it is to be misdirected, not because of a medical conspiracy, but because the institution of medicine is a human enterprise. Events like the Niacin debacle occur, is occurring and will recur. It is exceedingly difficult for medical studies to directly measure desired outcomes, such as living independently or keeping our wits about us longer. The desired outcomes are also called outcome measures and much harder to quantify. Medical studies typically measure surrogates, which may or may not correlate with outcome measures – important life events. Hopefully, surrogate markers are predictive, as studies can't always wait for life events to unfold. Researchers can only hope blood or imaging surrogate tests are good enough proxies or representatives of pathophysiology. Some examples include bone mineral density, (instead of bone strength), coronary artery calcification (instead of blood vessel plaque instability and narrowing) and erythrocyte (red cell) sedimentation rate (instead of inflammation). The Niacin Debacle, Keys' Cholesterol and the DREAM studies demonstrate the pitfalls of treating surrogate markers, and not the underlying disease. I wish to suggest that the focus on prediabetes and diabetes as an insulin deficiency is similarly misguided.

Establishing a line of causation, called pathophysiology is a moving target in medicine. When I studied pathology as a medical student, we were instructed to pay the least amount of attention to the pathophysiology section – it would soon be outdated. The last few decades have seen the blossoming of pathophysiology knowledge. Understanding of how the body functions (physiology) and fails to work properly (pathophysiology) has been expanding at an unprecedented pace. However, even as the science matures, maintaining skepticism is healthy, "Is this cause or correlation?"

One of the most interesting real life applications of this reasoning is the autopsy. Someone is dead; their body is on the table - that is the initial certitude. Can we establish with a high degree of certainty, from our understanding of pathophysiology, the sequence of events which led to their demise? Over the years, I had a nagging question about the most routine finding; almost a common incidental finding in almost every autopsy is atherosclerosis. Atherosclerosis links prediabetes-diabetes to the increased prevalence of heart attack, stroke, and most mental declines. Why do people still have atherosclerosis, albeit less frequently, even with near-normal blood glucose and lipid levels? Why do individuals who are declared healthy at their annual physicals by amiable doctors, silently harbor atherosclerosis at various stages?

The Insulin Resistance Theory

The key to answering these questions is insulin resistance. The insulin resistance theory plausibly ties the pathophysiology of atherosclerosis to hypertension, high blood lipids, chronic inflammation, obesity, diabetes, dementia and sedentary lifestyle. (Howard, 1996) Endothelial cells line the blood vessels, preventing clots while allowing nutrients to pass.

When their health is impaired, we have problems ranging from hypertension, clots to atherosclerosis. Endothelial cells become insulin resistant like any other cell in the body, resulting in high blood pressure as well as loss of the non-stick Teflon-like qualities. (Manrique 2014) It is no surprise that nicotine in cigarettes has been found to cause insulin resistance. (Bergman, 2012) Insulin resistance is highly likely to be the key to atherosclerosis. (D'Souza 2009 & DeFronzo 2010) Insulin resistance occurs in nearly all cells with insulin receptors: brain, liver, pancreas, and skeletal muscle, including the blood vessels lined by endothelial cells nurturing these organs. (Manrique 2014)

One of the earliest atherosclerotic change visible to the naked eye is a fatty streak, appearing on the inside lining of blood vessels, usually at a branch. Yellow fatty streaks taper, like a sink's rust stain from a leaky faucet. Over time, these streaks thicken, and bulge slightly, before becoming increasingly stiff plaques. Life is quite forgiving; until the next phase, most of these changes up to this point are completely reversible. These plaques expand to acquire an eroded sandpaper quality, burrowing into the vessel wall. The entire vessel wall gradually becomes rigid, fissured and brittle as the elastic stretchable membrane in the wall fragments. The roughened, now larger shard-like luminal surface juts into the bloodstream. Rarely the wall will suddenly fissure and balloon outward, forming what is called an aneurysm. More commonly, brittle fragments suddenly snap off, sailing like ice floes downstream. If the plaque fragment goes to the brain, perhaps a stroke or brief period of inability to speak follows, as a part of the brain is cut off from oxygen. Sometimes the plaque snaps open, like a trap door creating a sudden blockage which cuts off blood. Within a heart vessel, angina or a heart attack would result. If the blockage slowly narrows a smaller vessel, downstream cells gradually become strangled and quietly die slowly. It is common to see scars on kidneys – white, pie-shaped, depressed areas where sections have died off. The individual could have felt a twinge at the time or perhaps nothing at all.

Normal   **Fatty Streak**   **Complex Plaque**

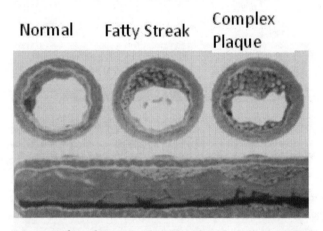

Years after leaving high school, I learned that my dear history teacher, who took smoke breaks between classes had suddenly died. Her daughter said to me, *"She looked fine. I don't know how this could happen."* I didn't have the heart to explain that atherosclerotic damage accumulates in blood vessels silently and invisibly. Sudden cardiac death is the largest cause of natural death in the United States, accounting for half of all cardiac deaths. Cardiac arrest can be the first time atherosclerosis announces itself. More shocking, atherosclerosis begins at an early age than most would guess. By late the twenties and early thirties, fatty streaks appear in the aorta, the largest artery in the body. Atherosclerosis is not merely a disease of aging.

Blood vessel damage is accelerated up to four times in Metabolic Syndrome and diabetes, even faster when fed by chronic inflammation such as in the situation of chronic gingivitis (bad teeth) or by smoking. Atherosclerosis only becomes apparent later in life, when enough damage has taken place.

The most commonly advised treatment or prevention of atherosclerosis is directed at surrogate blood lipid test levels, especially LDL (Low Density Lipoproteins) and HDL (High Density Lipoproteins). Maybe the reader is prepared to learn, a poorly known aspect of "bad LDL and good HDL" levels, is they are flimsy warranties against heart attack. Nearly half of all heart attacks occur in patients with "good" HDL and LDL levels. So why do half of patients hospitalized for coronary heart disease with "good" HDL and LDL levels have blockage of their heart vessels? (Sachdeva 2009). Clearly, HDL and LDL blood lipid profiles are incomplete surrogate markers of atherosclerosis. For us to devise a better treatment plan, a revised, more complete explanation is required. (Only partially "Fooled Again!")

The Insulin Resistance Theory is a mature, several decades old and well-accepted working medical theory which not only encompasses, but also is more comprehensive than either the Cholesterol HDL/LDL or Chronic Inflammation Theories. At the same time, the theory of insulin resistance causing disease is succinctly explains how elevated blood lipids and chronic inflammation act as partners in crime. So,

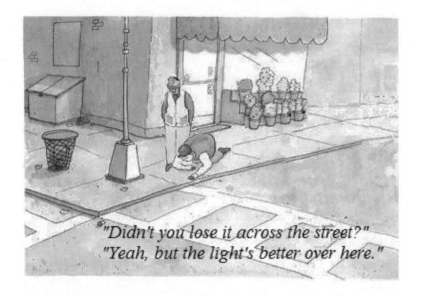

"Didn't you lose it across the street?"
"Yeah, but the light's better over here."

addressing insulin resistance addresses the most common cause of atherosclerosis as well as a host of other seemingly coincident but disparate diseases such as sarcopenia, hypertension and depression. Of these three, sarcopenia is probably the least familiar. "Sarco" means muscle. "Penia" means little. Together, Sarcopenia means "Little muscle," insufficient muscle, or "under muscled." Too often, sarcopenia is regarded as an inevitable part of aging – that's not inescapably so. All of these diseases are related, not just as cultural misconceptions of aging but also as co-conspirators in disease.

The Insulin Resistance Theory also explains why a dominant swath of the population silently develops the same suite of diseases, unrelated to atherosclerosis and blamed on aging. Please recall, physicians do not routinely order tests for insulin resistance. The diagnosis of insulin resistance requires active application of the Metabolic Syndrome inclusion criteria, first chart of this book. Because the hormone insulin not only regulates the glucose management of every cell, but also regulates protein and fat metabolism, insulin resistance causes widespread abnormalities. Take for example, central obesity – excess fat encasing kidneys, intestines and billowing out from an internal apron called the omentum. It's not possible to feel this internal fat by pinching the belly skin. These changes in our body are invisible to us without ultrasound, CT or MRI imaging. What is also called pear-shaped fat distribution, or to use more medical terminology, visceral (around organs), central fat has been found to be strongly associated with insulin resistance. Reduce extra central fat and insulin resistance decreases. Central fat is not subcutaneous fat, which is the fat which skin deep. "Pinching an inch" is the wrong focus when it comes to health. Reducing central fat through aerobic exercise can reverse insulin resistance.

Why Haven't I heard about Resistance Training for Insulin-resistance Before?

So if exercise directed against Insulin Resistance is the best treatment for the most common cause of atherosclerosis, why aren't daytime talk show hosts shouting it to their sedentary audiences? For me, I arrived at this realization only after several years of focused research. After The Niacin Debacle, I was not satisfied with answers from the most popular medical journals. Professional magazines often carry review articles to keep practitioners up to date. "Exercise is helpful for treating high blood pressure," or "Exercise is important for treating prediabetes." are typical exhortations seen from these publications. Most articles lack enough instruction to be actionable. Even if somewhat concrete, most healthcare providers are not in the best of shape or teachers of exercise as medicine. These vague statements probably mirror the advice of your provider, along that of my colleagues, as well as the advice of newspaper, internet and magazine articles. Many healthcare providers recommend walking because the compliance is relatively good.

Now and then, I began to follow-up on cited references from the Sports Medicine literature. This was the first time I had read scientific articles from this field. Like most physicians, I might not read more than one general medicine journal outside of my specialty. Reading journals from an almost boutique, niche specialty like Sports Medicine would be unheard of. Sports Medicine is associated with optimizing the performance of young athletes through training regimens. But that's not all. A sub specialty of Sports Medicine, called Kinesiology (not to be confused with Applied Kinesiology) specifically deals with strength and conditioning. Oddly enough, Kinesiology research tends to be better supported outside of the US, and so for both these reasons, doctors in training or in practice rarely if ever receive education in exercise as disease treatment. The two possible exceptions are Orthopedic Surgery and Physical Medicine and Rehabilitation (PMR). PMR assists patients recovering from accidents or coping with the effects of a debilitating disease. Physicians from both fields might read PMR articles and possibly Physical Therapy journals. Both of these fields use exercise, to help people with mechanical joint, muscle and tendon problems. Strength training doesn't fall into any mainstream field of medicine, so the kinesiology exercise research literature lies in obscurity in the US.

At least this is my explanation of why you might not have heard of strength training from your doctor. Since most doctors are taught to understand disease, not health preservation, this is understandable. Specialists might each have some parts of the knowledge in this book, but I have yet to know a doctor who will give specific exercise instructions. For instance, the endocrinologist who treats diabetics has extensive drug knowledge and some knowledge of diabetic pathophysiology – nonetheless a specific and useful prescription of exercise as treatment is a foreign concept. The cardiologist knows of cardiac rehab; the closest traditional medicine comes to using exercise to treat internal disease. And yet, cardiac rehab, which is a fancy name for aerobic exercise, while vital to repairing a damaged heart, is not often covered by insurance after hospital discharge. I once asked a PMR colleague, knowledgeable about exercise treatment of insulin resistance, why they don't publicize the treatment of Metabolic Syndrome or diabetes. He replied that they are busy doing physical rehab. Besides, he continued, they are a relatively small medical specialty without too much public presence.

It's Still Survival of the Strongest

Innumerable kinesiology and medical studies dating back more than 20 years have documented how physical DEconditioning (the opposite of exercise conditioning) is directly related to the decline of our metabolism. Although my specialty focuses on the mechanisms of diseases, I still found the strength of this connection a revelation. Pathology, the study of how things go wrong in the body is a five-year residency after medical school. Not once during residency, nor for two decades afterward, did I read an article connecting activity, muscles and atherosclerosis. Our culture tends to make the link less than obvious. Our sedentary, nonexertional lifestyle is designed to preclude strenuous muscular exertion. In the harsh environment of our ancestors, the physically strong were harder to kill. Now, our less powerful bodies deteriorate absent the need to fend off perils.

This manner of living causes the body's biochemistry to veer off from our evolutionary programming, like a rocket with a broken tail fin. Even less intuitive, relatively inactive muscles lead to a gummed up internal metabolic machinery. For those aware of Metabolic Syndrome and already in prevention mode, the main media message heard are dietary recommendations. Even those buying into the 10,000 steps walking program are missing the ancient requirement for recreating opportunities for intense muscle exertion. The vital message of exercise science research does not seem to receive equal exposure. Perhaps the research is not as home-grown, and has no large supporting professional organization; it also lacks a consumable product. Let's set aside now the social and cultural factors. In the next chapter, we will look at the intricate and fascinating fuel system of the body. We will see why "trying our best" is vital.

Chapter 3: Some pathophysiology: How things 'don't' work

Normal metabolism, before high insulin and glucose were the norm

The body maintains a remarkably narrow range of glucose between, during and after a meal as well as during periods when no food is being digested – too low, we feel lightheaded, too high, damages the body. The primary fuel, glucose needs active assistance, in addition to permission to enter cells. Insulin is the hormone which grants that permission. A host of regulatory substances such as incretins secreted by the gut, glucagon by alpha cells of the pancreas and a myriad of others play minor parts. It could easily take another detailed book to describe the entire physiological process, but this would distract us from the discussion. Suffice it to say, insulin is the director leading the orchestra.

Insulin receptors coat cells whose function depend on a measured fuel supply, the brain, adipose, skeletal muscle, blood vessels or measure fuel supply, the pancreas and liver. When an insulin molecule latches on the cell's outside receptor, cells heed an order to pump in the glucose and fat rushing by in the blood.

Consider the process at mealtime. (See the diagram below.) The liver, which is conveniently located downstream from the digestive or gastrointestinal tract, has first grabs at storing the incoming fats and glucose coming from a meal. The liver doesn't take in all the glucose. The pancreas, the body's glucose-thermostat sensor, monitors the rising tide of glucose in the blood, produces and releases insulin. Insulin signals to the body's cells to take up the fats and glucose. So when glucose is flooding in from the gut after a meal, healthy individuals rapidly clear blood glucose with the help of baton-waving insulin. Some of this glucose goes to the liver, but in healthy people with a normally functioning glucose-insulin system, 70–90% of glucose will be stored as muscle glycogen. (Knuiman 2015) After the meal is neatly stored in the liver and muscle, the remaining are packed away into long-term fat stores. The pancreas gradually cuts back on insulin production as glucose and fat are put into their proper places. Glucose levels fall to premeal levels. A lab test of how well this whole system functions is the Glucose

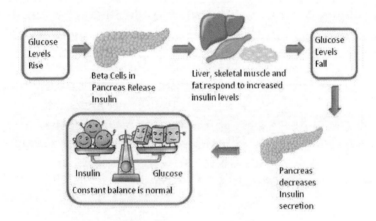

Tolerance Test (GTT).

Between meals, the liver stabilizes blood glucose concentration within very narrow limits by dispensing glucose from previously stored liver glycogen. Glucose is released proportionally to insulin levels, which in turn is regulated by the pancreas. The liver is the sole source of glucose released into the fasting bloodstream; without it, we would be hypoglycemic between meals! The liver also functions as an energy currency exchange. Sugars can be changed into fats and proteins morphed into sugars. The liver can continuously match the body's fuel needs as required. For example, when the liver's glycogen levels are depleted, after a prolonged period of not eating, fat stores are tapped for energy. Here again, insulin instructs fat cells when to release stored their fat. The liver reprocesses available fuel stores, gradually releasing precisely what the body's tissues require during this fasting period. Fasting blood tests, drawn before the morning meal, principally measure how well the liver is performing this function. The fasting blood sugar (FBS), measures how well the liver's performance when it comes to glucose.

The third most common test for glucose handling is the Hemoglobin A1C test. The glucose sugar attaches to the hemoglobin molecule. That attachment accelerates at higher levels of glucose. Red cells which contain hemoglobin, last about three months before being recycled. Hemoglobin A1C makes an excellent test for the average level of glucose over 120 days. To recap, the three most commonly used tests for diabetes, test three different aspects of glucose-regulating ability or insulin resistance. The FBS measures the liver's ability to manage fasting periods; GTT, the body's ability to handle meals and the Hemoglobin A1C, the long-term average.

In preparation for the next level of discussion, please briefly reread from the beginning of this section. See how many places insulin acts and imagine the aftermath, should insulin's interaction go awry. When you are done, let's move onto what goes wrong.

Metabolic Syndrome has its roots in insulin resistance

Diabetes is a combined abnormality of insulin production and signaling strength. Type 1 diabetes from the onset is a problem of inadequate insulin production, which is due to the own body's attack on the insulin-producing, Beta cells of the pancreas. Think of it as fratricide. Meanwhile, Type 2 diabetes, prediabetes and Metabolic Syndrome begin with insulin resistance. The cause of insulin resistance is not insulin, nor an immune reaction as in Type 1 diabetes, but a cell's insulin unresponsiveness or deafness. While "Insulin resistance" might seem to be shrouded in mystery, scientists understand the mechanisms of insulin resistance to the molecular level. Our discussion needn't delve so deeply. Knowing both Type 1 and Type 2 diabetes patients develop insulin resistance, we can devise exercises to reverse the process and benefit both forms. Insulin sensitivity or its converse, insulin resistance is not difficult to understand, once explained.

Consider loud music, the deafening kind you might have liked when you were young. When a live concert begins, the music volume is overwhelming. But by the time that the opening band finishes their set, the noise level sounds comfortable. Your ears have become desensitized to loud music. By the time you leave the concert, normal levels of sound are hard to hear. You might be unknowingly shouting at your friends on the drive home. Without too much repeated abuse, your ears can recover by next day. Go to too many Grateful Dead concerts and you become a Deadhead or Ear! Insulin's target cells are like your ears, and insulin is like the loud music. The cells have become desensitized to insulin. Insulin resistance begins at a low level and with time gradually increases. The initial event might be nicotine from smoking but in most cases, lifestyle is to blame. (Bergman, 2012)

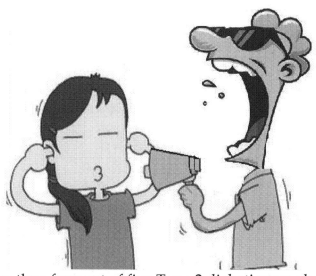

More than four out of five Type 2 diabetics are obese in the US. The fat surrounding the abdominal organs is thought to cause insulin resistance. (Hardy 2012) In the conundrum of lean Asian diabetics, it appears to be a deficiency of muscle and sedentary lifestyle. (Sattar 2015 & Misra 2008). In both cases, insulin resistance starts in the with either central fat deposits and/or poor quality and relatively small muscles. A very small portion of adults develop Type 1 diabetes after early adulthood. We will examine the science behind the exercise to address both of these types of insulin resistance is later in the book.

In the overwhelming majority of cases, insulin levels start out slightly elevated in Metabolic Syndrome peaking prediabetes, before declining later in Type 2 Diabetes, This condition termed hyperinsulinemia, simply means elevated insulin levels. Likewise, when elevated blood insulin levels are abnormally high relative to glucose levels, it's diagnosed as insulin resistance. Insulin resistance indicates that it takes a higher concentration of insulin to achieve the same level of glucose. Hyperinsulinemia is an abnormal physiologic state with negative consequences. Studies have clearly demonstrated hyperinsulinemia in seemingly healthy and active people acts like poison. For example, in 1971, 1326 policemen in Helsinki were tested for abnormally high insulin. Looking back, after 22 years, researchers found hyperinsulinemia accounted for heart attacks, "independent of other cardiovascular risk factors, including blood glucose, cholesterol, triglycerides, blood pressure, indexes of obesity and its distribution, smoking, and physical activity." (Pyorala 1998) Since then, studies expanded to women, have added to the mounting evidence that hyperinsulinemia in outwardly normal people, with otherwise normal lab levels is damaging. (Rewers 2004) The Insulin Resistance Atherosclerosis Study showed a strong association between hyperinsulinemia and thickening of the carotid artery wall, an early sign of atherosclerosis. (Howard, 1996) Translated into common English, insulin resistance can account for atherosclerosis, masquerading for changes wrongly blamed as aging.

Under ordinary circumstances, a doctor will not order insulin levels to diagnose insulin resistance. The diagnosis of insulin resistance is made clinically, by applying the criteria for Metabolic Syndrome. So having one or more of the criteria, including a BMI >25 for Caucasians and >23 for Asians is reason to have a GTT, FBS or Hemoglobin A1C test. The common denominator in Metabolic Syndrome, high blood pressure, prediabetes and diabetes is insulin resistance. While many prediabetics will not progress in their lifetime to diabetes, the diagnosis of a high glucose test value or the criteria of Metabolic Syndrome is a call for action.

Let me give share this analogy for insulin resistance. Suppose someone has rented a low-powered, putt-putt, subcompact without cruise control and is driving across the Midwest. Unbeknownst to them, there is a headwind that blows constantly and increasingly stronger the farther west they drive. The radio is blaring as they try to maintain the speed limit. At one point, the driver realizes that they have dropped below the speed limit. Looking down, they notice that the pedal is flat on the floor. The overheating, little car engine is beginning to issue white smoke. Our subcompact has just been diagnosed with prediabetes. Its engine (the pancreas) unbeknownst to the driver has been valiantly trying harder and now is beginning to fail. The headwind or insulin resistance caused by central fat or deconditioned muscle has been getting all the while stronger. The overheated engine has begun affect the rest of the car (our body) by overheating the radiator and fraying the drive belts. For the longest time, we just assumed it was the car just getting old. If our car was broken down awaiting a tow truck, we'd be in the diabetic phase.

On the Road to Diabetes

Let's take a conceptual look at the three phases of Type 2 diabetes. Early on, insulin is able to keep pace with insulin resistance, so that if we were to only measure glucose, it would seem as if nothing is amiss. This is like the gas pedal slowly making its way to the floor to keep the speed up in an ever increasing headwind. Only after the pancreas' insulin production begins to petter out, glucose begins to rise.

Conceptual Progression of Prediabetes to Diabetes Disease Course

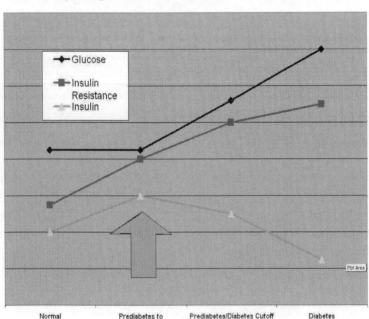

Hyperinsulinemia is present long before glucose rises.

People just diagnosed with prediabetes are not in the first inning of a baseball game. They are at the top of the fourth inning, up against last year's pennant winners, scoreless and behind. Many people mistakenly think an elevated fasting glucose level (more than 100 mg/dL) is the first stage. Glucose does not begin to rise, however, until after the pancreas has started to capitulate, and by that time, the problem has already been brewing for years. The pancreas has been trying, unbeknownst to us, to put out higher insulin levels in the hopes of driving down glucose. In spite higher insulin levels, the organs increasingly turn a deaf ear and like drug addicts, in their diseased state say, *"I want more, and more insulin to do the same job!"* This goes on over time until the pancreas says, *"Uncle! I can't put out any more insulin. I'm exhausted!"* After that breaking point, glucose levels begin to rise, eventually into the diabetic control range. So while it is not possible to know who will progress to full-blown diabetes, insulin resistance is what must be avoided, before the stress on pancreatic Beta cells results in their demise. (Berman 2002)

The window for reversibility lasts roughly eight years and begins to close after the period when the pancreas reaches exhaustion. (Knowler 2009) The longer the interval before the primary problem is unaddressed, the less time remains for it to be reversible. Clearly, catching insulin resistance before attaining the prediabetics phase is best. Most physicians will refer prediabetic patients to dietitians and recommend some exercise. Dietary advice and aerobic exercise are the most common and standard care diabetic "lifestyle changes" recommended. "Talk is cheap," and studies prove that out. (Sharma 2008) Studies of the effectiveness of dietary advice rank just about zero. Effectiveness increases in the following order: Diet plus exercise advice, diet plus exercise classes and diet plus exercise classes totaling more than 150 minutes per week. Structure matters.

Weight loss, especially of central fat, will reverse the insulin resistance. Being able to "Pinch an inch" of belly fat is the wrong focus. Recall that it's not the fat just under the skin that is the more dangerous of the two. While in many cases, aggressive weight loss will be enough to reverse insulin resistance, experience has taught us that, in many cases, hard-earned diet-induced weight loss has only been a futile delaying action. After a few years, the problem of rising glucose recurs. The pitfall can be avoided by dealing with all of the causes of insulin resistance.

With rare exception, *every Metabolic Syndrome, prediabetic and Type 2 diabetic has some relative ascending degree of insulin resistance.* The principal correctable problem in our control is insulin resistance. Insulin resistance is not only the result of central fat, but also poor quantity and quality of muscle. If the liver becomes insulin resistant, it will release excess glucose overnight. As a result, the fasting blood glucose (FBS) test will be high. If we were to measure insulin levels and multiply that by glucose, people with Metabolic Syndrome would have a higher than normal product, called an insulin Disposition Index. In other words, the higher the Disposition Index, the more likely someone will eventually become diabetic. (Lorenzo 2010)

Measure of Insulin Resistance Disposition Index = glucose x insulin level

For a moment, consider this equation from a treatment standpoint. Halving insulin resistance halves the required insulin level. Changing insulin resistance means that prediabetics can revert to a normal state, and diabetics can potentially preserve their Beta cells. The Beta cells of the pancreas don't die from overwork. So how can we decrease insulin resistance for the better?

On days we're not exercising, the brain, kidneys, liver and the intestinal tract together account for three-quarters of demand for glucose. Between meals, these organs steadily take up and use the glucose coursing nearby in the bloodstream. At mealtime, the liver isn't the only organ taking up the mealtime outpouring of glucose, fats and proteins. Likewise, the liver isn't the largest glucose storage depot. By far, the biggest potential home for a meal's glucose is skeletal muscle. Skeletal muscle can take up a staggering quantity of glucose, a minimum of four times the storage capacity of the liver – even more for those with larger muscles. For glucose, it is a one-way ticket into the skeletal muscle, to be stacked like cords of logs, ready to burn for the next major (not minor) exertion. Unlike the liver, muscle cannot release glucose back into the bloodstream. Until a relatively high exertion level is experienced, the muscle's glucose and fat sit, awaiting the call. For many who are sedentary, or who exercise only with only minimal intensity, that call almost never comes – which we'll learn later on, is a bad situation.

Muscle is the most alterable organ in the body. With the proper exercise prescription, it is possible to change not only the amount of muscle, but also the quality of the cellular machinery and in turn, tune-up the entire body's physiology. The first time that the plasticity of muscle/muscle's plasticity became evident to me was when first watching the 1977 documentary *Pumping Iron*. This entertaining, not to be taken seriously, yet enlightening vignette, shows monstrous male models in bikinis lift weights, and modify (as well as show off) their bulky, but trained muscles. In an outlandish manner, Arnold Schwarzenegger and company show how resistance exercise can make muscles larger -- in medical terms, hypertrophic. In one memorable scene, they examine each other, pointing out muscles and suggesting exercises to improve their prominence. Increasing muscle size is not rocket science. Not as obvious however is how responsive muscle can be to prescriptive exercise. With much less strenuous exercise, muscle can be trained to demand more than 85% of the body's glucose and make it a sink for circulating fat. While we can't easily control the liver's overproduction of glucose, we can change the absorption of glucose and fat through exercise. The secret which I haven't let on until now, is muscle controls fat and glucose metabolism and bigger muscles control metabolism even better.

Larger muscles soak up more glucose: Creating a welcome home for glucose

Generally speaking, people who have more muscle can tolerate a much higher caloric and carbohydrate meal because they have more muscle tissue mass to store the glucose outpouring from the intestines. Earlier in the book, we noted that Asians get diabetes, even when they are not overweight. In addition to central fat cells triggering insulin-resistance, insufficient and poor quality muscle trigger insulin-resistance. This subtype of Type 2 diabetes, called *lean* Type 2 diabetes occurs in relatively low BMI people, regardless of their ethnicity. They suffer from low pancreatic insulin production coupled with declining skeletal muscle mass of inferior quality. Think of someone who is relatively scrawny, vegetarian, living that office-to-couch lifestyle or bizarrely enough, even that avid runner. (Everaert 2011, Baguet 2011) Asians share this relative sarcopenia, developing diabetes at a BMI >23. Most Asians born in the last century did not have an adequate protein intake, resulting in stunted muscle bulk. Unlike the Western diet which is plentiful in meat, Asians substitute vegetarian proteins which lack certain key amino acids, which yield far fewer Type II muscle fibers. Inactive middle-aged citizens of the US develop an analogous muscle problem – a double whammy of ebbing muscle bulk later in life through inactivity coupled with poorer quality. Asians start off with fewer Type II fibers, and develop diabetes at a lower BMI as a result of meat-protein poor, childhood diets. We'll discuss more about muscle fibers in a short while.

Muscle has an under-recognized role in metabolism, especially when discussing the metabolism of food, far more important than the Glycemic Index (GI). Glycemic index is the idea that foods have different absorption rates. Blaming simple versus complex carbohydrates or the Glycemic Index of food is yet another misguided concept. Foods with high Glycemic indexes are said to be absorbed quickly and jolt or cause blood sugar to spike up. Studies of Glycemic index also are unable to take into consideration the mixing effect of different foods and their glucose handling. (Augustin 2002) Another misconception is that the intestine is a passive organ, filtering fuel into the bloodstream – this is too simplistic an understanding. A set of hormones known as incretins communicates with the pancreas as well as other organs to smooth the absorption and processing of food. Indeed, the pharmaceutical industry has taken the opportunity to create a whole class of drugs influencing incretin behavior, such as exenatide (Byetta, Bydureon), liraglutide (Victoza) but to name a few. These drugs mimic the natural amplification role incretins play in calling up insulin. As a practical matter, trying to manage diabetes from a digestive angle is simply a sideshow to the main event. In the same way, modifying diet by eating low Glycemic Index foods to control diabetes has little, or no demonstrated long-term benefit. Whether the Glycemic Index in practice can control diabetes is highly questionable. The underlying problem in Metabolic Syndrome or diabetes is not the Glycemic Index load of a meal, but the aberrant way that the body processes the meal as the result of insulin resistance. Eating small meals with slowly absorbed calories does not fix the underlying problem of insulin resistance, the cause of diabetes.

It should be no surprise inactivity has an effect on the single most changeable organ in fuel-processing –

skeletal muscle. For our predecessors, not more than three generations ago, daily life was a continuous strenuous and demanding exercise. Rarer were the times when one had the luxury of resting and conserving energy. Those were precious moments for them. Who knew when they would suddenly flee or be called upon to pitch in? Compound that lifestyle with the uncertainty of the next meal. The body needed to store long-term energy, (fat) whenever the opportunity presented.

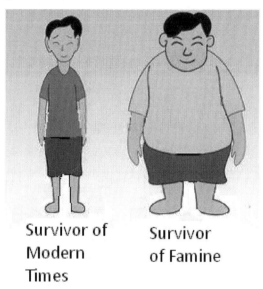

Survivor of Modern Times

Survivor of Famine

We are descendants of the fat storers

Even a magazine from the supermarket checkout line will tell us that diabetic control can improve through weight loss. Sure, losing fat through dieting decreases insulin resistance, but almost immediately, this strategy runs into a roadblock. First the body fights back, releasing hormones which scream, "I'm hungry, gorge me whenever food presents." After about a day, the body enters a catabolic phase problem for those who attempt to lose weight through aerobic exercise and/or low calorie dieting. Remember, eons ago, famine genetically culled those who could survive. We are the descendants of survivors of famine. Over millennia, this natural selection means storing fat when times are fat. This catabolic phase of metabolism therefore brings us to experience the time-tested, life-saving metabolism which served our ancestors well during lean or starvation times as a weight loss plateau. Catabolism prepares our bodies to survive the proverbial crop failure or long winter, sacrificing to hang on, until bountiful times. When the body switches to a calorie penny pinching, i.e. catabolic mode, it becomes increasingly difficult to lose weight. Lean times dictate hormones like insulin which govern metabolism are in a self-preservation mode. People who are obese already have high circulating insulin levels which resist touching fat stores – the reason why overweight individual have a much harder time losing weight. As anyone who injects insulin for Type 2 diabetes knows, insulin spurs weight gain. So at some point, initial pounds that fell off easily, hang on tenaciously as if survival still depends husbanding fat cells.

Is there no wonder why dieting feels exhausting! Catabolism is not the direction we want to travel for another reason; the body begins to resort to self-cannibalism, avoiding protein building, and in cases trimming down protein structures that it doesn't deem necessary. The body sees inactive, high-maintenance protein muscles and says, "I don't need to replace these muscle fibers anytime soon and certainly don't need to make more." Look at pictures of T-Rex's grappling hooks; they look like the arms of professional road bike cyclists, rail thin without much muscle. Even their cyclist-like bodies don't see much use for arm muscles. In the same way, the yo-yo weight loser gets a double whammy – less muscle and more fat after regaining that original weight level. A diet plus aerobic exerciser, or just dieter will lose 25% muscle for each 75% of fat. (Dengel 1994) Typically the diligent dieter will fail around the time of family gatherings or Thanksgiving holiday. The holiday weight rebound tends to not contain muscle, and so re-achieving the same weight level is attained with less muscle than ever before. (Beavers 2013) Less muscle means translates into the same weight, but lower basal metabolic rate.

Just as adipose tissue is a repository of fat for the body, skeletal muscle is the ready storehouse of protein amino acids. The body needs proteins on a constant basis, to replace the worn down levers and gears of machinery. Skeletal muscle functions like a protein warehouse. Muscle composes about 75% of all bio-available protein in the body. It has among the highest turnover rate among organs, breaking down and building proteins continuously. Intense exercise increases the turnover rate and in turn, metabolic rate. Said another way, exercise breaks down muscle and requires protein to rebuild muscle fibers. The process of rebuilding muscle requires more energy than simply having more muscle! This is just one more reason why inactivity leads to weight gain, and why the resistance exercise can help.

Of the three macronutrients, (micronutrients are those

required in small quantities such as vitamins and metals) carbohydrates, fats, proteins, proteins are the hardest to synthesize and most prized, like a gold watch that we work hard to get. And when times are hard, fat and glucose easier to convert into energy. While the body loath to pawn protein for energy, protein can easily be converted into fuel energy. Cutting calories for weight loss added to perceived minimal use of muscles, such as steering a bike handlebar, however leads to loss of muscle.

In the heavy meat consumption countries of North America, Western Europe and some other countries, Type 2 diabetes is associated with obesity. As a result, many erroneously believe that obesity and more body tissue simply overwhelms and overtaxes the pancreas, so it cannot produce enough insulin. Likewise, in the minds of many practitioners of medicine, the paradigm of diabetes treatment surrounds weight reduction by any means. Even while this theory retains a kernel of truth, the concept is at best incomplete and results in the poor public health situation. While especially important for the obese, weight loss works primarily through reversing insulin resistance by reducing central fat, only one of two major mechanisms of insulin resistance.

For those overweight, losing weight especially in the early stages of diabetes or prediabetes sometimes is sufficient for returning blood glucose to a lower or normal level. Many may know this process as the familiar idea of "eating less" or "eating right" and aerobically "exercising." A person weighing 185 pounds burns 356 calories per hour at walking speed and 450 calories per hour at a jogging pace. Assuming a pound of fat has 3500 calories, it would seem to take 8-10 hours to lose a pound of fat, right?

Wrong! (Sorry, had to throw you a trick question to demonstrate the value of correctly framing the issue.) The reason is simple. Recall, diet and aerobic exercise lead to 75% adipose loss and 25% protein (muscle) loss. This type of weight loss method loses muscle. Multiple studies, including a 2011 study by Kristen Beavers' group at Wake Forest University reveal the unwitting muscle loss with aerobic exercise and dieting. According to the study, the major protein reserve in our body is skeletal muscle. (Beavers 2011) In turn, basal metabolic rate is largely dependent upon the amount, turnover of skeletal muscle and lean body mass principally determines the basal metabolic rate. Skeletal muscle, when taken in conjunction with the proportion of adipose tissue, accounts for the basal metabolic rate. (Wolfe 2006) Researchers can predict an individual's new, adjusted basal metabolic rate by taking into account the new weight and new total muscle mass. Unless one keeps or increases skeletal muscle mass during dieting, basal metabolic rate will decrease. This is why diet plus exercise leads to weight plateauing.

Diet plus aerobic exercise = muscle loss = decreased basal metabolic rate

Burning off calories for weight loss through dieting or aerobic exercise only partially solves the problem of basal metabolic rate. Although diet and aerobic exercise do well and are most commonly advised in treating Metabolic Syndrome or prediabetes, studies have shown that either dieting, or aerobic exercising, or both together will not stop the majority from progressing from prediabetes to diabetes. (Xiao 1997) A well-regarded and scientifically backed group of scientists and doctors now believe the solution is to change the focus to building muscle tissue through resistance training combined with aerobic exercise and eating a healthy, nutrient and protein dense diet. (Hawley 2004, Davidson 2009, Church 2010, Dijk 2012, Winett 2014, Earnest 2014)

The *principal problem cannot be fixed without addressing muscle insulin resistance and increasing basal metabolic rate.* Only proper exercise can correct the underlying insulin resistance caused by skeletal muscle. It is not sufficient to simply reduce the mass of adipose tissue. Properly structured exercise can rebuild, rewire and reprogram the metabolic muscle machinery. Now you have a full understanding we have not been using all of the tools in our armamentarium to combat Metabolic Syndrome to diabetes. Resistance exercise cultivates one organ in particular: skeletal muscle. Think of the three as a prescription – only that type you don't get in a blister pack with aluminum backing.

I won't rehash what constitutes a sensible diet, but not because it isn't important. Call it my greenish desire to conserve trees. I suggest the DASH diet (Dietary Approaches to Stop Hypertension) as a starting point. I will have more to say about protein, in a later section.

Strong muscles give glucose a home: Reverse insulin resistance

Almost everything you will read or hear about glucose

control will barely mention resistance exercise. But the US Health and Human Services, American Diabetic Association, American Heart Association, American Sports Medicine Association and many others recommend resistance training, in addition to aerobic exercise, and diet as the three cornerstones to combating diabetes and the precursor prediabetes. We've mentioned my personal theories as to the reasons resistance training remains unemphasized if not underemphasized. This section is the "meat" of the book where we'll share muscle's role in aging and diabetes.

Physiologists recognize underutilized muscle becomes disused without strenuous exercise. In other words, an undemanding, modern lifestyle causes a diseased muscle which directly leads to an abnormal metabolic state. For most, physicians included, how our well-fed, nutrient complete diet can lead to diseased, debilitated muscle, which in turn leads to a host of metabolic diseases is far from obvious. As alluded to earlier, splitting up the problem into ones of quality and quantity can be helpful. Muscle plays a vital, almost unknown and under-recognized role in metabolic health. Most people in developed economies suffer from muscle disuse. Over time, unchallenged muscle becomes insulin-resistant, which is relatively small, poor in quality, and impaired by sticky stagnant fat and disused sugars. As a result, cellular enzymes which regularly handle the lion's share of metabolism become deranged. When these defective muscle enzymes are presented with fats and sugars to process, they set in motion a pathologic chain of events. And when the problem is compounded by an inclination for Type II muscle fibers to shrink with time and inactivity, the scope and quantity lead to widespread mayhem. Let's breakdown the sequence of events.

Sarcopenia, a clue to fixing the metabolism

We often think of skeletal muscle as this dumb, mechanical organ which unpretentiously contracts. Additionally, some might know that muscle produces heat, explaining why seniors feel colder at the same temperature or why sitting still can feel cold. Science in the last two decades has learned of many more roles. For instance, contracting muscles secrete hormones called myokines. Among many myokine functions, we know that some act like attractants to stimulate nerve ingrowth, others coordinate metabolism between organs, keep the heart healthy, boost the immune system, improve endothelial cells, and relax blood vessels, perhaps even help kill early cancer cells as well as a myriad of other functions. (Pederson 2011) For decades, epidemiologists have known of tantalizing connections between dementia, reduced cancer, better heart functioning, and exercise, but up until the discovery of myokines, science had no mechanism to explain the phenomena. Muscle does much more than contract. We will explore but one of these little-known roles with insulin. (McLeod 2016)

We mentioned earlier that elevated glucose could be divided into two time periods. While we sleep, essentially fasting, the liver persists in putting out glucose even when insulin is signaling "stop." The other during the daytime, and by far the longer time, is when glucose is inadequately absorbed by smaller, sarcopenic, inactive muscles. Both instances, when glucose levels are persistently high, glucose turns into a troublemaker. This elevated glucose is like a band of rowdy wayward teenagers who are bent on making mischief, eventually taken in by central adipose tissue or randomly attaching to proteins throughout the body. In the first instance, the liver converts glucose into circulating fat in the form of triglycerides. High blood triglycerides in turn, are stored in fat cells or cause mischief in nonadipose cells. In cells, the delinquent glucose molecule gums up our body's enzyme and proteins by latching on to tool-like proteins, interfering with their normal folding and ability to speed chemical reactions. One test measuring the phenomenon of glucose's attachment to protein, the hemoglobin protein molecule, is the Hemoglobin A1C test. What's happening to hemoglobin, is happening to proteins all over the body. To see one common example where glucose's and fat's attachment messes up the functioning of metabolic machinery, look no further than the endothelial cell. The blood vessel lining cell's enzyme machinery is wrecked by these toxins, preventing normal relaxation of wall tension, resulting in high blood pressure.

I always think of sarcopenia, whenever someone brags, "I weigh the same as when I was in my twenties," implying this somehow means they are just about as healthy. However, by "watching what one eats", or exclusively doing aerobic exercise, our bodies will gradually and inexorably lose muscle, year after year. Although youthful, but out-of-fashion clothes still fit and the scale below seems to indicate no change, Superman's x-ray vision would see a very un-Superman-like decline. With a sedentary lifestyle, the average person will lose an astounding 50% of muscle mass over a lifetime. That's displacement of muscle with fat, roughly 1% annually after age 30. Look at the elderly slowly walking or struggling to get up from a chair. Among cyclists, the first sign is slower speeds when climbing hills. Sarcopenia leads to lagging reflexes, weakness, falls, fractures, dementia, and an inability to continue with an active lifestyle.

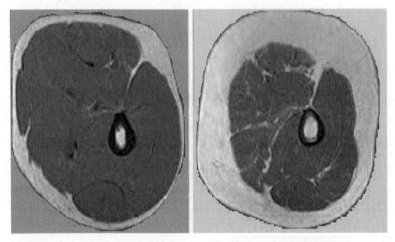

Let's take an inside look at the legs that can still fit into those pants. These are MRI cross sections through the leg of a young person (left) and a person about 60 who is relatively inactive (right). The dark portion is muscle and the light part is fat. The center black circle is the femur bone. Take a moment to compare how each part has changed. Muscle doesn't turn into fat as some might fear. Rather, unused muscle shrinks in size and is displaced by fat, sometimes lending the same outward appearance.

Personal experience can be just as convincing without an MRI. Around the late 40's to 50's most people notice their metabolism slowing down. Some might attribute "hormones" to this problem, or, for women, "menopause." Mostly, however, this is a direct effect of having less skeletal muscle mass over time. Researchers have conclusively found that the slowing of metabolism is directly proportional to the decrease in total muscle mass. Less muscle and less actively rebuilding muscle equates to a slower metabolism. Sarcopenia, the gradual loss of muscle mass, equally applies to the earlier enigma of weight loss plateauing.

This age-related change, sarcopenia is fascinating at the microscopic level. Every muscle in the body, except for the muscles controlling the motion of the eye and vocal cords is a hybrid of two muscles. Microscopically, with special staining techniques, this hybrid resembles a patchwork mosaic of Type I and Type II muscle fiber bundles. Type I fibers are aging resistant, so called slow twitch fibers. These muscle fibers operate with a different set of metabolic machinery than Type II and are strengthened by aerobic exercise. (Martin 2000) Type II fibers are aging sensitive, so called fast twitch fibers and are responsible for generating greater strength. Type II fibers are reserved for heavy loads. Let me restate this in another way. Type I fibers can take care of themselves overtime. Type II fibers need nurturing. Without regular heavy challenges, Type II fibers will naturally become smaller with the passage of time.

Fiber Type	I	II
Contraction Speed	Slow	Fast

Fiber Type	I	II
Strength	Weaker	Stronger
Aging Resistance	Excellent	Needs nurturing
Energy Source	Aerobic	Anaerobic

At the root of nearly all insulin resistance is relative sarcopenia of Type II muscle fibers and Type I to a less extent. Nearly all people who do not regularly expose themselves to strenuous muscular challenges will have some degree of Type II muscle fiber sarcopenia, which only worsens over time. Obese individuals may be carrying more weight, but are proportionally under muscled. Type 2 diabetics are generally corpulent with proportionally larger than average muscle size, but that muscle has been shown to be metabolically-poisoned, dysfunctional skeletal muscle. (Ciaraldi 2016) Stagnant glucose has latched onto proteins within the muscle cell, inhibiting their function. Fat molecules which have overstayed their welcome, are transformed into rancid, crazed signaling molecules, which wreak widespread organ havoc.

In the muscles of active children, and under normal conditions, glucose is taken out of the bloodstream, repeatedly replenished and stored by the boatload in muscle. Skeletal muscle glucose is stored as a glycogen with a glucose storage capacity more than four times that of the liver, even more with activity. Both the liver and muscle take glucose in from the bloodstream and piecing it together in a regularly branching, beautiful, 3D structure resembling the ornamental plant, Silver

Mound, called glycogen.

What does glycogen that stores adjacent to contracting muscle fibers do? The muscle stores glycogen as a ready-access, high exertion, energy source. For very short bursts of energy, say 15 seconds or less, muscle relies on Creatine Phosphate, a kind of flash-in-the-pan, flashbulb energy source. After a bright burst kick starting muscle contraction, Creatine Phosphate's power is gone, and so to keep going, skeletal muscle uses glycogen. Super-efficient, sustained fuel from when our ancestors needed to get out of trouble quickly, glycogen in skeletal muscle is the primary fuel source when the intensity of muscle contraction is above 50% of maximum. This is when Type II fibers are required. Those who are unaccustomed to exerting themselves will never touch this glycogen storehouse, leaving it stagnant, like a pond cut off from an intermittently nearby flowing stream. As a result, the muscles never experience an ongoing need to be topped off by glucose during meals. We'll have more to say about this later and see how the same happens with muscle triglyceride fat stores.

Chapter 4: Toxins and Stagnant Ponds

Poisoned muscles

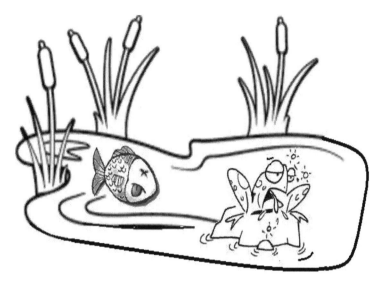

Glucose stagnates and thereby insulin-resistant muscle is severely impaired in taking glucose and fat out of the bloodstream as well as storing it. This inability is the other major cause of insulin resistance other than fat. The roughly 15% of Type 2 diabetic patients who are not obese develop insulin resistance exclusively from inactivity and sarcopenia. These so-called "lean diabetics," or "sarcopenic diabetics," are most prevalent among especially among Asians from India and Pacific Rim countries. This typical person is 50 years of age, thin, not firm, maybe a little sagging in places. Their childhood was characterized by a low meat, possibly vegetarian diet. Their muscles have a lower proportion of Type II muscle fibers because low animal meat diets are deficient in certain amino acids. In all other respects, their Type 2 diabetes is similar to overweight diabetics. If they have been regularly lab tested, their fasting glucose and triglyceride have been slowly inching up, and HDL going down over the preceding decade. (Misra 2015)

Obese and nonobese diabetics have similar muscles. Biopsies, or small thigh muscle samples typically show the muscle cell is failing to do its metabolic job. (Ciaraldi 2016) The inactive muscles suffer from the effects of rancid fat and stagnant glucose toxins, which researchers have called glucolipotoxins. Glucolipotoxins are the fat and glucose molecules accumulating in muscle, endothelial, brain, liver and fat cells around internal organs. Glucolipotoxins are responsible for transmitting metabolic dysfunction throughout the body's systems, resulting in the constellation of disease associated with diabetes.

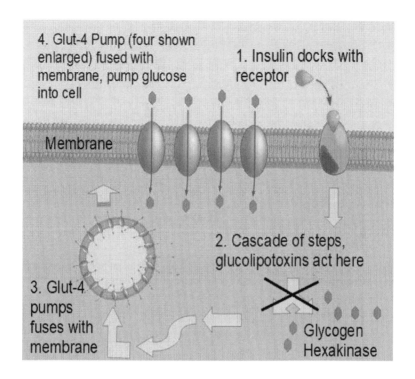

4. Glut-4 Pump (four shown enlarged) fused with membrane, pump glucose into cell

1. Insulin docks with receptor

Membrane

2. Cascade of steps, glucolipotoxins act here

3. Glut-4 pumps fuses with membrane

Glycogen
Hexakinase

Muscle Insulin Resistance at the Cell Level: Glut-4 Glucose Pumps

Researchers have a relatively good idea of how glucolipotoxins cause insulin resistance. I'll give you a short description on this now and later, the rest of the astounding story. Insulin resistance doesn't have anything directly to do with the hormone molecule insulin, nor the docking port, where insulin attaches to the outside of the cell. On the inside side of the cell membrane, docking is supposed to activate a cascading series of enzymes, like a set of arranged dominoes. In the final step of this process, a sac full of glucose pumps called GLUT-4 moves upward to the surface of the cell membrane. The sac then fuses with the cell membrane and the GLUT-4 pumps glucose into the cell. The problem lies between the docking and fusion phases, where glucolipotoxins have poisoned intermediate enzymes. The enzyme cascade peters out, preventing the GLUT-4 filled sac from moving as well as the enzyme (glycogen hexokinase) that pieces the glucose molecule to the beautiful, Silver Mound-like, glycogen spiral chain. It turns out that muscle cells have a backdoor to release this faulty mechanism, but you will have to read on.

Circulating Fat chance

So far, you have only heard the half of the story about insulin resistance that pertains to glucose, not fat. Physicians tend to focus on LDL, downplaying the importance of triglyceride levels, since they are not an independent risk factor for heart or vessel disease. In studies, triglycerides levels are not as statistically as strong an independent risk factor for heart attack or stroke, when compared with LDL or HDL. That's why triglycerides have lost center stage. Ask some physicians and they will say that triglycerides only become important when very high (500 mg/dL). At this level, triglycerides can lead to pancreatitis. Other diseases cause elevated triglycerides such as genetic disorders, Nephrotic Syndrome, chronic renal failure, hypothyroidism, alcohol, high carbohydrate intake, tobacco use and medications. While, on the one hand, elevated triglycerides are the result of numerous factors, on the other, fish oil, especially the enteric-coated variety, can lower triglycerides. Fish oil contains the well-known omega-3 fatty acids docosahexaenoic acid (DHA) and eicosapentaenoic acid (EPA), which lower triglyceride levels]. Keep in mind, however, I am not suggesting omega-3 fatty acids as a way to resolve the problem of elevated triglycerides. There are limits to supplements, to prescription and nonprescription interventions, as well as to your ability to self-diagnose underlying causes for your condition. After all, high triglyceride levels in certain diseases are surrogates, rather than bad actors, so lowering them might not be the most efficient treatment. To get a better sense of your specific needs, consult your medical provider.

Instead, I would like to call attention to the role triglyceride as a barometer for insulin resistance, and the first laboratory signal of progression toward diabetes. Doctors know that diabetes control correlates well with triglyceride levels. For insulin resistance, triglyceride levels are like the canary in the a coal mine mine shaft— they are the first warning sign that something is out of balance in the body. The steady rise in triglyceride levels precedes all other tests suggesting increasing insulin resistance, even fasting blood glucose. Since we don't routinely measure insulin levels, the unhappy canary of insulin resistance might manifest as years of rising triglyceride levels. The lab values of progression are insulin levels, triglycerides and finally glucose. Remember insulin levels top out before glucose rises, so high glucose levels are a late sign in a chain. Those who keep personal medical records might wish to take the time to compare their triglyceride levels over time. The direction in which these numbers change can give a good indication of whether insulin resistance is developing.

According to studies done on those of European

descent and Koreans, the ratio of triglycerides to total cholesterol is a good marker for insulin resistance. A few studies suggest that a ratio of 2.75-3:1, triglyceride to HDL predicts insulin resistance in men and >1.65 in women (Cordero 2008, Kannel 2008) Other groups have not been studied to establish an exact worrisome ratio.

How has your canary been feeling lately? "Rising triglycerides levels may indicate increasing insulin resistance"

Elevated fasting triglyceride levels not only are a sign that metabolism is worsening, but also are considered by some to be the problem underlying diabetes. Triglycerides are a subset of circulating fatty acids; triglycerides are stored in adipocytes (aka fat cells) and serve as an important energy source during conditions of fasting and exercise. In people with a healthy metabolism, triglycerides should fall within hours after eating meals.

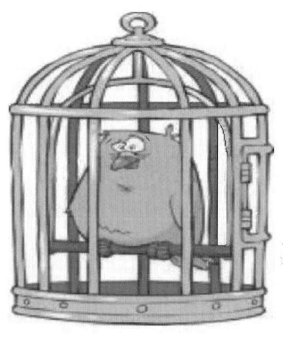

Aside from glucose, insulin regulates fat as well as protein transport in and out of cells. An under recognized action of insulin is the signal it gives adipocytes to store fat. High insulin levels prevent adipose tissue from regressing. Overweight people have higher insulin levels as a consequence of central fat induced insulin resistance. High insulin levels, whether from injections or from insulin resistance, prevent weight loss, yet another problem for those with obesity related Type 2 diabetes. Treatment of weight loss must be therefore directed toward reducing insulin resistance. Recall from our discussion of the Disposition Index that small changes in insulin resistance cause reciprocal changes in insulin levels. Decreasing the Disposition Index by decreasing muscle insulin resistance allows insulin levels to naturally fall and helps considerably in making loss of fatty tissue easier.

Treating both muscle and adipose tissue insulin resistance, it is possible to break the negative feedback loop which eventuates in diabetes. Together, both high levels of circulating fat and glucose inundate cell insulin signaling pathways and result in insulin resistance.(Corcoran 2007) Researchers have called this "lipotoxicity" recognizing fat's role as a toxin, in addition to glucose. Evidence identifies "lipotoxins" and glucotoxins as acting together as glucolipotoxins that "poison" the Beta cells of the pancreas, cells lining blood vessels, brain cells and muscle cells. Since all cells in the body use energy, no cells are seemingly immune. The cells lining blood vessels become susceptible to atherosclerosis and high blood pressure with insulin resistance. (Manrique 2014) Chronically elevated blood free fatty acid and glucose concentrations are thought to cause widespread glucolipotoxic damage to brain tissue and nerves. Unsurprisingly, scientists have linked insulin resistance to dementia and exercise to its prevention. (Ma 2014)

Evidence that accumulation of fat in liver results in particularly severe damage is a condition known as fatty liver. Teetotalers and many diabetics develop a condition called fatty liver. In the former case, the toxin was high dose alcohol, in the latter, glucolipotoxins. In this condition, the liver turns from a dark mahogany brown to a yellowish light tan. Regardless of the cause, with a microscope, it is easy to see the color change is the resulting accumulation of fat droplets within liver cells. With the epidemic of obesity, diabetic fatty liver now ranks as the third most common cause of cirrhosis in the United States.

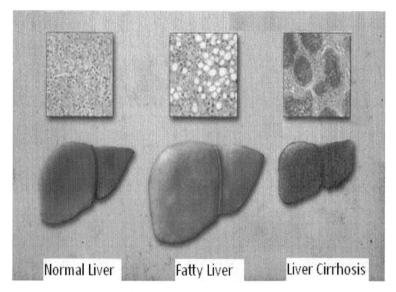

Normal Liver   Fatty Liver   Liver Cirrhosis

An intriguing drug side effect demonstrates how muscle, especially the type of muscle produced by strenuous activity might help clear blood lipid levels. The first-line cholesterol-lowering class of drugs called statins [(atorvastatin (Lipitor), lovastatin (Mevacor), pravastatin (Pravachol), rosuvastatin (Crestor), simvastatin (Zocor)] has an unusual and uncommon side effect of muscle pain and weakness. This reaction occurs in about 1 in 10,000 patients taking a statin, (although some believe it to be far more common.) Researchers discovered patients with the side effect have antibodies to HMG-CoA, the enzyme responsive for manufacturing cholesterol in the body. Patients have soreness because the antibodies attack muscle cells, especially the newly minted, regenerating muscle cells which have even more HMG-CoA! (Longo 2016, & Mammen 2011) So muscle cells and especially new muscle cells have more enzymes devoted to handling fats!

The other aspect that could reveal the role that muscle plays in fat metabolism is a more common side effect of statins–tipping borderline prediabetes patients into diabetes. This risk increases with higher doses and with duration of statins. Nonetheless, medical authorities still believe that the benefits of statin therapy outweigh the risk, so please don't change your prescription based on this information. (Anastazia 2015) As an aside, evidence supports CoQ10 supplementation may prevent the rise of glucose caused by statins. (Mabuchi, 2007)

I have listed these examples to make the point that muscle is an unsung hero when leading the way toward reducing glucolipotoxins throughout the body. Muscle can clear glucolipotoxins, absorb excess glucose and fat from the bloodstream and through resistance exercise, breakdown, discard old toxin-damaged proteins and manufacture untainted ones. Rehabilitating muscle can lead the rest of the organs in ending the vicious cycle of insulin resistance.

Your muscle is like a Prius, a hybrid vehicle

My Toyota Prius drives in all-electric mode below 10 mph. Above 10 mph, the gasoline engine kicks in to help. Some Prius owners who want bragging rights to extreme gas mileage, try to keep below 45 mph. Above these speeds, the Prius' gasoline engine is continuously running with an occasional acceleration boost from the electric motors.

Your muscle's fuel management system is like the Prius drive system, using different fuels at different speeds.

At low exertion levels, less than 30% of maximum, muscles draw fuel from the bloodstream. At moderate exertion, from 30-60% they use some glycogen and blood glucose in addition to muscle-stored triglycerides. At the mid and higher levels of exertion, the liver recycles expended energy packets in a process called the Cori cycle or lactate pyruvate pathway to assist the exercising muscles. That's why high levels of exertion result in huffing and puffing. Above high-moderate exertion levels, 60-70%, they significantly dip into muscle glycogen stores and requiring help from all sources to keep up the demand. (Knuiman 2015)

People who don't exercise hard, are always in the lowest third power mode, the Prius' all electric mode. These people are the couch potatoes and the walkers. Their muscles aren't accustomed to switching into a higher fuel mode. While this takes fuel from the liver

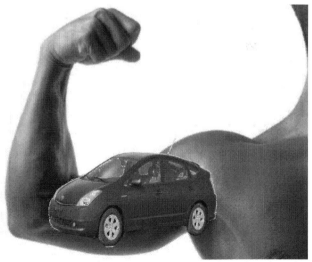

glycogen stores and fat to reduce weight, this method is

woefully inadequate to prevent sarcopenia.

The middle zone includes endurance exercisers, like joggers, who manage a steady pace for 30 minutes, five times a week for the recommended 150 minutes a week. These middle tier exercisers, are like the Prius' most efficient mileage mode for eeking out the most miles per gallon. Their muscles are seldom accustomed to switching into the highest mode. Recall that aerobic exercise stimulates Type I muscle fibers which are already aging resistant. Those Type II fibers are not getting any longevity boost!

Only those who perform either moderate or high-intensity aerobic exercise or the twice-a-week resistance exercise can teach their muscles new tricks. Confusing intensity with duration is common. Exercising to 55 to 85% of maximum heart rate is an example of important, sometimes ignored aerobic exercise intensity recommendation.

For aerobic exercisers, we can summarize as follows. At low levels of exercise intensity, most of the fuel is coming from bloodstream sources outside of the muscle, from liver glycogen and from some fat stores. At moderate levels, more fat stores are being used, so this is a more efficient zone for losing weight than the lower zone. For reversing insulin resistance, a higher intensity is needed. Only in the upper half of intensity, does the muscle begin to draw from energy sources from within the muscle. Utilizing muscle's internal stores of energy with enough intensity is therapeutic. Only by driving down the muscle's stores can one seek to flush out stagnant stores of fat and sugars. Repeatedly replenishing muscle fuel stores creates healthy adaptations.

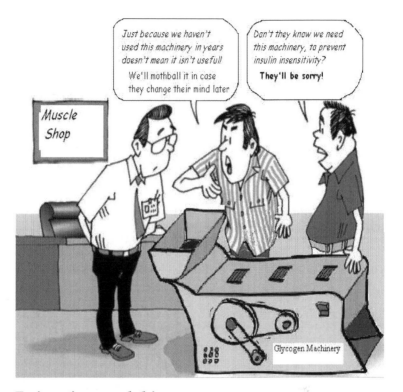

Fatigue is a good thing

In order to get the most metabolic benefit it is important to exercise muscles until exhaustion. With exhaustion, comes added metabolic bonuses of muscle adaption, increased number of blood vessels, increased power-generating units, fat dissolution, and renewal of youthful cellular machinery. Furthermore, exhaustive exercise repeatedly draws down and rebuilds muscle glycogen reserves. Intensely drawing own or recycling, for instance, causes the muscle to release anti-inflammatory, hormonal, and possibly brain building substances.

A desired result of repeatedly drawing down glycogen muscle stores is increased insulin sensitivity. Exercising muscle to exhaustion encourages muscle to request more glucose, each time making glycogen stores slightly larger. Muscle cells can then adapt by increasing the number glucose transport receptors (GLUT-4) on the cell surface to accommodate the perceived need for more glucose. (Cartee 2015)

In the absence of resistance training, unused muscles get pared back, especially Type II fibers. Fast reacting muscle fibers shrink with time. Fewer nerve endings attach to the muscles. Even the metabolic cell machinery gets decommissioned. When these unused systems go offline, our metabolism suffers. As much as we might try to remain blameless and blame slowing metabolism on aging, research clearly shows otherwise. Studies show, however, that the process is reversible with effort. The cell machinery inside the muscles can be cleaned up, lubricated and restored, especially when it comes to handling fat and insulin.

This redrawn diagram illustrates a skeletal muscle trick which no other body organ can replicate. With vigorous or strenuous contraction, a previously insulin resistant muscle converts into an insulin receptive muscle for about a day, maybe even two. Luckily, exercise has a signaling pathway which runs parallel and cross talks with the previously blocked insulin-signaling pathway. So after exercise of sufficient intensity, the insulin receptor becomes primed for about 36 hours afterward to handle meals more normally. Even if the muscle cell has been insulin resistant, the insulin response will revert to a responsive or sensitive state during this time, huge boost to our body since exercising muscle can be the largest consumer of fuel.. (Koopman 2005 & Hawley 2008)

Intense exercise increases the muscle's insulin sensitivity by spouting more GLUT-4 receptors making GLUT-4 channels become once again abundant. (Maarbjerg 2011) These changes do not occur at "no

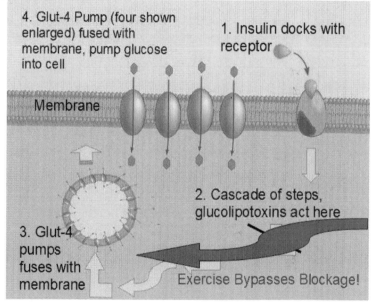

4. Glut-4 Pump (four shown enlarged) fused with membrane, pump glucose into cell

1. Insulin docks with receptor

Membrane

2. Cascade of steps, glucolipotoxins act here

3. Glut-4 pumps fuses with membrane

Exercise Bypasses Blockage!

sweat" levels of muscle training. Reversing insulin resistance has precisely the effect sought in a diabetes drug. Imagine if pharmaceutical firms could package into a pill what exercise can achieve by reversing insulin sensitivity, they would have a blockbuster drug. But you can have it without going to your local pharmacy, simply by exercising correctly!

I wish to add a fine but important point on the need for intensity in exercise. We can look at intensity from both an aerobic versus anaerobic standpoint as well as from a muscle fiber viewpoint. Let's consider aerobic first. Endurance exercise is aerobic by definition; one can exercise for an extended period of time without stopping. If aerobic exercise is of moderate or lower intensity, muscle draws fuel from predominantly from the fat stores because body fat has the largest energy stores in the body and aerobic metabolism of fat is highly efficient. As a result, exercising aerobically for a long time is best for fat reduction, but is not the same as exercising more intensely. Aerobic exercise in the higher half or highest third intensity level also uses energy fuel stores in the muscle itself. So only a sufficiently high Type I, aerobic muscle fiber exertional intensity, can reverse muscle insulin resistance in Type I fibers.

Sufficiently challenging anaerobic resistance exercise achieves the same effect for Type II fibers. Intensity in this circumstance doesn't mean getting out of breath or achieving a certain heart rate. In order to revert Type II fiber's insulin resistance, intensity means lifting to fatigue. Studies have shown identical results whether fatigue is achieved by lifting lighter weights many times or heavier weights fewer times. As long as the last repetition can't be performed, performed while preserving correct form, you will have achieved that necessary level of intensity. This has been termed exercising to "momentary failure". It is a scary term, but doesn't mean lifting dangerously. It simply means to do your best. For both aerobic or anaerobic exercise, the metabolic goal is to make the muscle feel fatigued.

In our sedentary modern society, the reduced level of

intensity, duration and frequency of exercise has resulted in an inadequate recycling of glycogen and triglyceride stores in skeletal muscles. As a result, persistently high fat and blood glucose, cause other organ tissue and blood vessels to become gradually insulin resistant. Over time, high levels of circulating glucose and fat (glucolipotoxicity) damage nerves, muscles, pancreas, blood vessels and other tissue throughout the body.

Most people have seen under-exercised muscle, but cannot recognize it. You can see for your own eyes next time when visiting the meat counter; take a look at the most expensive steaks. Fatty rivulets marble premium steaks such as Filet Mignon, New Strip, or Porterhouse. Although these cuts are admittedly tasty, if these steaks are representative of the muscles inside your body, they 'cost' you dearly in terms of metabolism and are functionally poor muscle. Fat and stagnant sugars inside muscle like these high priced cuts contribute to insulin resistance and poorly functioning heart muscle in chronic heart failure. (Haykowsky 2014) Whether in a cow or inside us, these muscles can only be cleaned up by intense exercise.

Strong (and sore) muscles can fix your lipid problem!

Let's examine the reasons why exercising to exhaustion for aerobic exercise should be your metabolic goal. To begin, I find making a distinction between the source of energy to be helpful. Glucose versus fat are the two major choices for energy. Other fuels exist, but are not central to insulin resistance. Glucose and fat as fuels are compartmentalized within the muscle (intramuscular) and outside the muscle (extramuscular). Recall glucose and fat are toxins as well as fuels, so these have a dual nature and targeting intramuscular stores, play a role in reversing insulin resistance. Insulin resistance, in turn is the result of poisoned enzymes. Enzymes like any structure in the body are are continuously recycled, the rate is determined by demand. If we can induce new production, then any subsequent fresh batch of enzymes won't be tainted. Therefore, the purpose of exercise is to induce turnover of the intramuscular fuel/toxins. A relatively high threshold of exercise intensity determines whether this occurs, because only at a high intensity does the overall fuel mixture or balance between glucose or fats usage tilt in our favor.

When exercising at a low intensity, 30-65% of maximum effort, circulating fatty acids from extramuscular sources are primarily being burned, the proverbial fat burning zone. People whose primary goal is to lose weight, generally exercise at 60% of maximum heart rate. However, only at a higher level of exercise intensity, does the switch to burn down muscle fat and glucose stores get flipped. So in order to reverse insulin resistance, the stagnant sources of glycogen or glucose as well as fat intramuscularly, or within the muscle need to be turned over. Without cycling down intramuscular glycogen, it is not possible to significantly reverse insulin resistance. The muscle cells will then sense a higher calling. Muscle cells adapt by dusting off the unused machinery, maybe unused since your childhood – cell fuel management systems which reverse insulin resistance.

Take a look at the chart below which summarizes visually what we shared. In 1993, Dr. Johannes Romijn demonstrated that certain metabolic muscle machinery doesn't get turned at low levels of exercise intensity. (Romijn 1993)

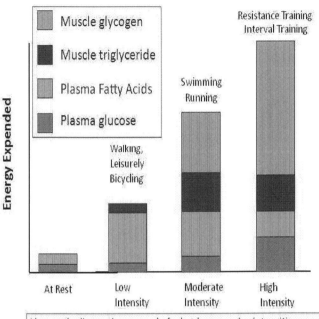

Liver and adipose tissue supply fuel at low exercise intensities. Muscle fuel and machinery are only used at high exercise intensities.

You may be familiar with some terminology associated with lifting weights. Often times trainers talk about sets and reps (repetitions). One set might consist of ten repetitions. After ten, perhaps the muscles feel tired and are unable to complete another repetition. That is called a "ten repetition set."

We feel muscle fatigue when the glycogen stores are depleted in the contracting muscles. The glucose in muscle is insufficient to activate calcium release necessary for orderly contraction. An experienced cyclist climbing a hill, intuitively know how to manage muscle glycogen to the top. At the top of the hill, glycogen reserves are almost exhausted. (That's why I always say, "Hills are your friends!" to my hill-adverse, two-wheel compatriots.) After about two minutes of relative rest, glucose from the bloodstream will restore sufficient glycogen – to allow renewed activity. The larger the muscle exercised, the more exhausted the muscle, the more glucose and fat will be drawn down from the within the muscle stores.

When performing a high-intensity muscle contraction set to fatigue, the muscles draw down glycogen from muscle stores – like a rechargeable battery. Only when glycogen levels reach a low level do we experience fatigue. At this point, muscle glycogen goes into a temporary deficit, and it takes a little time to recharge. With larger loads, both muscle fiber types are utilized to meet high energy requirements because all hands are needed on deck. (All galley rowers or if you prefer, the Prius is in combined electric and gas mode). Not just Type I fibers, but also Type II fibers require to rebuild glucose stores. Glucose from glycogen stored in the liver and triglyceride-like fatty acids from fat from adipose tissue stores are released into the bloodstream. Glucose and fatty acids are then absorbed from the bloodstream by all muscle fiber type cells.

When we are couch potatoes or if we limit ourselves to walking, even slow jogging, those glycogen stores are rarely drawn down and re-topped off. We find ourselves with a problem our cave-dwelling ancestor's bodies probably only rarely encountered. With glucose circulating in abundance, muscle glycogen stores brimming within muscles, where does all that glucose from a meal go now? When do the tainted machinery get replaced with brand new ones? The body is loath to waste any of excess fuel and the glucose gets stored as fat. The liver takes excess protein and makes it into glucose. Excess glucose is transformed into fat. The fat, or blood lipid floats in the bloodstream until it is taken up by fat cells.

Take another look at Dr. Romijn's chart above. Can you see that the green (muscle glycogen) isn't touched by muscle during low-intensity exercise? If muscle glycogen remains untouched during exercise, skeletal muscle will mothball rarely used cellular machinery over time. The green part, (the top two rectangles which appear only on the moderate and high-intensity bars) or the glycogen stored in each muscle, is the largest store of glucose in the body. If not drawn down with regularity, the pancreas will need to increase insulin levels to send it elsewhere. The goal in combating insulin resistance is to employ as many of the large muscles to burn down glycogen. For many sedentary friends, the largest and poorest conditioned muscles are in the low back. Consequently low back exercises are part of the recovery process. Making space for glucose makes life easier for the pancreas. Reactivating insulin sensitivity by energetically exercising the biggest muscles is the most efficient manner to reverse insulin resistance.

Chapter 5: All exercises are not the same, the sum is greater than the parts

Two different muscle fibers = two different exercises

Although aerobic and resistance exercises are different exercises for muscles, most dynamic muscle contraction exercises fall within a spectrum from resistance to aerobic. Exercises employing numerous repetitions with no or light resistance fall into the aerobic category. To illustrate this point, let's do a thought experiment. I grip a traditional resistance exercise, two-pound dumbbell and do what is called a biceps curl by flexing the biceps muscle. Although the biceps curl is a traditional resistance exercise, using an exceedingly light weight, transforms the curl into an aerobic exercise. For myself, I can easily perform 100 or more repetitions before boredom would cause me to stop. At a low demand physiologic level, the biceps muscle contracts with fuel supplied from the bloodstream, without becoming short of oxygen. The biceps muscle is not sufficiently challenged enough to be at the highest intensity level – not from a fatigue nor exertion standpoint. More resistance load is required before the exercise can be called a resistance exercise. Curling a feather-light, hand-held, barbell repeatedly throughout an hour-long TV show is an example of a probably minimally effectual, aerobic exercise with a token amount of resistance.

Aerobic exercise traditionally has been somewhat misconstrued as almost exclusively a heart-lung enhancer. While the heart does strengthen with this type of exercise, the aerobic benefit mostly accrues to rest of the body. Aerobic exercise in truth, improves aerobic respiration, in other words, primarily the aerobic metabolism of muscle. So while the heart and lungs do experience some improvement, the majority of aerobic exercise enhancement occurs elsewhere at the skeletal muscle cell level. Specifically, the muscle cells become more efficient in using oxygen.

Therefore, if speaking of increasing the fuel efficiency of muscular motion, endurance, we are talking about Type I muscle cells which have an oxygen optimized – also called aerobic or oxidative – fuel system. Type I cells are aerobically efficient as the result of possessing

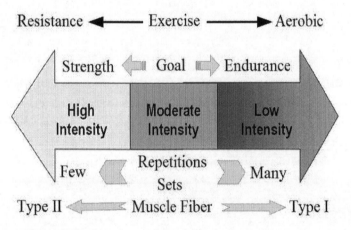

more energy power plants – called mitochondria. While mitochondria are in all cells, the transformational improvement throughout the body with aerobic exercise is headed up by muscle cells. When you are huffing and puffing, muscles feel "short of breath", they adapt in several ways including making more mitochondria and growing more blood vessels. The muscle cells also lead the way forward to better health by releasing myokines which signal to other cells the need to get more fuel efficient or restated, get more work done with less oxygen. Metabolically, the last two changes are synonymous.

The Type I fiber, aerobic system's design sacrifices lean fuel efficiency for strength. Imagine for a moment the archetypal long distance runner – svelte and sinewy, little fat not unlike a famine survivor. Alone, Type I fibers barely have enough strength to bear minimal loads, a system designed to help us survive starvation. Prior to the 20th century, daily survival depended upon a supplemental, powerful, yet relatively fuel inefficient – anaerobic system which is called upon only when more strength is demanded. That parallel system would be the Type II fiber.

When an exercise calls for more strength or if a few repetitions result in fatigue, this exercise falls into the category of resistance exercise. The equipment type, such as a barbell does not determine the muscle fiber type exercised. For instance, a weight heavy enough to perform up to approximately up to twenty more repetitions is resistance exercise, if more than 20 repetitions can be performed, then the effect on muscle is aerobic. A heavy a weight load exceeds a muscle's sole reliance upon the bloodstream to sustain oxygen. When muscles forcefully contract, compressing blood vessels, no additional blood-borne nutrients can reach the muscle cells, including oxygen. For example, if you have painted a ceiling, then you know it's much harder keeping your arm overhead, compared to painting the wall. Oxygen-deprived muscle cells respond by augmenting anaerobic enzymes. These beneficial changes only occur at high resistance when Type II fibers become engaged. In other words, the muscle when challenged in this way, feels "inadequate." Type II muscle fibers increase strength, by awakening sleeping stem cells, which in muscle are also called Satellite cells that begin to multiply. Satellite cells can increase the size of muscles at any age. (Wang 2012)

Aerobic and resistance exercise promote complementary Type I and II fiber adaptations. Using both types of exercise, upgraded muscles and other cells work more efficiently. A more efficient muscle equates to accomplishing the same workload with less fuel or oxygen. As a consequence, the heart doesn't need to pump as rapidly. Many accredit a low resting pulse rate to a stronger heart when in fact, it is mostly a sign that the body is more conditioned, tasking the heart with a smaller metabolic load. Exercise, especially high-intensity exercise cleanses away stagnant metabolites, by increasing the flux of glucose and fat. Renewing cells produce untainted protein enzymes which in turn create a cleaner metabolic slate. In this manner, aerobic exercise reverses insulin resistance for Type I cells, while resistance exercise reverses insulin for Type II muscle cells.

The Fick Principle

Here is an analogy for a low resting pulse rate. A small electric motor (the heart) turns a belt that is tied to a heavy grindstone wheel (the metabolism). The grindstone is required to turn at a certain minimum speed at all times. If the grindstone wheel is taxing for the motor, the motor will heat up, especially when the grindstone sharpens a big object. If a stronger motor is swapped in, it can turn the grindstone with ease, perhaps not even heating up. If the grindstone axle, representing our metabolism is oiled, or the grindstone loses some weight, through exercise, the motor experiences even less stress. This is a well-established link between resting heart rate and metabolic efficiency. Physiologists have named this relationship

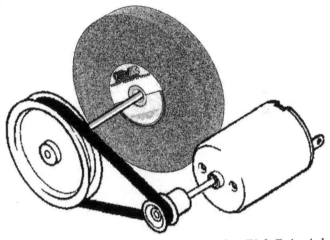

between the heart and metabolism, the *Fick Principle*.

Exercise improves the grindstone more than the motor, by creating an aspiration for the body's cells to be better. We know this because of the two, higher intensity is far more effective compared to longer duration of exercise. The most effective aerobic exercise is high-intensity, short time, interval aerobic exercise. "High Intensity Interval Training" (HIIT) has a progressive aspect which is a cut above traditional endurance aerobic exercise. We won't delve too deeply, but HIIT shares an instructive aspect with progressive resistance training. *Signaling the need for improvement is the purpose of exercise.* HIIT is exercise of very short duration, so HIIT does not work directly, but rather induces physiologic change. Just like progressive resistance training, HIIT is the stimulus that triggers a desired aerobic metabolic response. The body feels inadequate, "not up to task" and subsequently adapts in response but only after the exercise has ended. Low intensity walking can only be a stimulus for nonwalkers. After achieving a certain level, only a stronger stimulus can trigger subsequent adaptations. As an aside, HIIT studies performed with diabetics have shown impressive benefits, as well as a time-efficient way to achieve similar if not superior results. (Little 2011)

Whether challenging the muscles with heavier weights or higher exertional levels, the nervous system increases the number of nerve connections in a process called muscle recruitment. When muscle is called upon to lift a heavy load in resistance training, fibers are called up in sequence of metabolic efficiency. The aerobic Type I fibers get the initial call up, followed by the Type II anaerobic fibers. Likewise, centrally aligned fibers get the call up before more tangentially aligned fibers. (Heinonen 2012) The progressive call to action, over time increases the number of nerve connections, which in turn leads to faster reflexes. Without resistance training, this muscle fiber recruitment gradually declines with slowing reflexes.

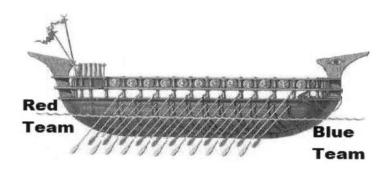

Red Team

Blue Team

Nerve-muscle recruitment is responsible for a large increase in strength. Imagine a two-tiered galley with Red Type I fiber rowers and Blue Type II fiber rowers. The Red Team Rowers sit closer to the water, always have their oars in the water never fail to row. Over time, the Blue Team Rowers decided not to row as hard because the coxswains, (the motivational guys with whips or hand-held bullhorns depending on your century) had gradually quit calling on the Blue Team Rowers. Turns out, the Blue Team Rowers became lazy, because when the call came to row, the Red Team Rowers had already gotten the ship moving. Only when the captain wanted to go faster did he call upon the Blue Team Rowers to row. Eventually, the captain gradually stopped calling upon the Blue Team Rowers because he lost the desire to make the galley sail fast. Recruitment is like waking up the Blue Team Rowers and hiring more coxswains. The captain needs a way to attract more coxswains, in other words, muscle stimulating nerves.

If you are past 30 and don't strength train, not all your muscle fibers respond when you move a heavy object.

You must wake up and reconnect with the Blue Team Rowers by lifting heavy weights. When this happens, muscle fibers entice the nerves to grow outward by secreting a myokine attractant called Brain Derived Neurotrophic Factor (BDNF). At the time of this writing, a myokine connecting skeletal muscles to the brain has yet to be discovered. However, it assuredly exists as intriguing exercise studies show a simultaneous rise of rising BDNF levels within the brain. This could explain why exercise is associated with new neurons in the brain, and a concurrent positive effect on memory and mood.

Professional athletes, whether they are baseball players, football players, or cyclists know resistance training is the most time-efficient way to develop the largest, strongest and most responsive muscle. I'm assuming that few among us are professional athletes, but weight training doesn't discriminate. It will work for professional or amateur, old or young, thick or thin. Training muscles is an ongoing process, so the amount of weight resistance that one chooses to begin with doesn't matter. What matters is progression – a commitment to continuous progress. Since weights can be incrementally adjusted, the degree of challenge to muscles likewise can be calibrated. Muscles are among the most malleable of the body's organs. We only need to raise the bar when challenging muscles for a continuous improvement in size and quality. Incentivizing the muscle means that the challenge we present to muscles never stagnates. We'll tie continuous improvement to the concept of progressive resistance in the later chapters.

Resistance and aerobic exercise upgrade our capabilities in different ways. Research has conclusively shown that together, resistance paired with aerobic exercise is far superior to either alone: Waist measurements, blood pressure, insulin resistance and triglyceride control all improve. The take home message is that resistance training added to aerobic exercise are superior to either alone. Indeed, many studies share this "two are better than one" mentality." In a landmark study of markers of Metabolic Syndrome, researchers discovered combined exercise had the best results when triglycerides, blood pressure, waist measurements or HDL were measured. (Bateman, 2011) The findings have been confirmed in other subsequent studies. Don't short change yourself by doing only aerobic exercise or a semi-aerobic-strength training class.

Sometimes I get a question about about yoga. In theory, yoga as an isometric exercise should also be considered a form of body weight resistance exercise. Some studies have explored its potential role in treating Metabolic Syndrome, prediabetes or diabetes. While some studies show promise, the low level of scientific quality limits drawing firm conclusions. No rigorous, high-quality scientific studies have been performed to date.

Chapter 6: Weight loss is the wrong focus

What should be the focus?

It's commonly known that loss of just three to seven percent of excess weight can lead to improvement in insulin resistance. For reasons that are not yet apparent to researchers, the loss of central body fat, as opposed to the fat underneath skin (subcutaneous fat), greatly improves insulin resistance. As a result, many people are told to focus on weight loss to improve glucose control. While weight is a convenient measure, by now you should know that skeletal muscle has been missing from this discussion. Without addressing muscle, regain of central fat is almost inevitable. So what matters is body composition, the relative proportion of quality muscle to fat. Weight is a secondary consideration. Those wishing to improve metabolism need to focus on improving the quality and quantity of skeletal muscle mass (also known as Lean Body Mass) and decreasing central fat.

It's not a big step to realize the popular BMI (Body Mass Index) calculation while handy, is hardly the best measure of health. Indeed, the early 19th Century inventor of BMI had little training in nor understanding of physiology. A trained economist, Adolphe Quetelet classified populations with his knowledge of mathematics and statistics. He created BMI as a broad demographic measurement in sociology and criminology for what was known as Social Physics. Perhaps most curious, the father of BMI, never intended BMI to be a measure of individual health. In fact, more accurate as well as simpler measures of health such as the ratio of height to waistline exist.

One of the best quality of life predictors is total skeletal muscle, otherwise known as Lean Body Mass. Less total skeletal muscle mass is associated with lower quality muscle, less strength and early loss of mobility in later years. (Visser 2005) Muscle is our primary, ready reserve of protein storage in the body. When the body needs to repair damaged tissue, protein comes from the diet or muscle. Healthcare workers know a burn victim's survival correlates with their total skeletal muscle mass. Healing of the skin and soft tissue draws upon this muscle protein reserve, determining the speed of healing.

The elderly often live on the knife edge of sufficient muscle mass. Compensation for decreasing strength begins in midlife with labor-saving devices such as elevators. Our culture of automation has inexorably reduced the demands of daily living. Over the last century, daily caloric expenditure has dropped such that mundane challenges to exert oneself have been innovated away, to the detriment of our metabolism and muscle mass. As a result, prematurely frailty has been unwittingly facilitated by modern technology. With barely sufficient muscle reserve the elderly might be hospitalized for elective surgery or unexpectedly after a fall. The required prolonged bed rest immobilization further weakens the muscle, tipping them into a "catabolic crisis," from which they may not recover. Building and maintaining a generous protein reserve (muscle) can be lifestyle saving as well as lifesaving.

Squaring the Curve

Aerobic exercise is strongly associated with prolonged

lifespan. Population studies performed on a theoretical 45-year-old suggest an incredible 7:1 return on bonus lifespan for each minute spent aerobically exercising. (Moore 2012) Once when I suggested eating healthily to a patient, she jokingly retorted that abstaining from her favorite foods would only make life *seem* longer! Many would ruefully agree that the total number of years lived doesn't matter as much as the quality of time – resistance training plays a role here. By increasing total skeletal muscle mass, one spends a longer time enjoying independence. We demonstrate this phenomenon by "Squaring the Curve." Please take a look at the "Squaring the Curve" diagram below. Aerobic exercise might establish the final tail of the curve, but resistance exercise pushes the curve up and to the right. Where the curve intersects the horizontal "independent" line largely depends on the quantity and quality of skeletal muscle mass.

Anabolic Resistance: Why you need more protein

Adding and maintaining skeletal muscle mass is more difficult, but not insurmountable for older adults. The young teenager and twenty-some-year-old can stimulate muscle protein growth just by eating protein. After about 60 years of age, **both** resistance exercise and eating a higher protein diet are required to stimulate muscle growth. This blunted muscle building response is termed "Anabolic Resistance." (Philips 2014) While Anabolic Resistance is a well-recognized phenomenon especially for those with cancer, the underlying mechanism is still the focus of intense study. Pending future discoveries, we do know as far as sarcopenia is concerned, increasing protein intake, possibly with an emphasis on branched chain amino acids, the type found in whey supplements, can help greatly. In other words, at this age, insufficient protein intake is often the cause of poor muscle strength gains and this can be overcome as easily as adding a supplement.

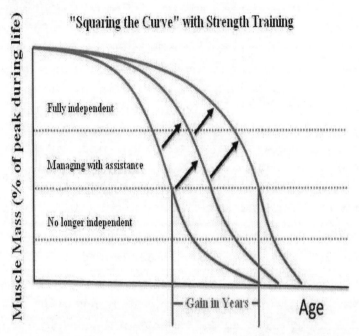

Successful resistance training gains may require more than the present RDA universal dietary recommendation of 0.8 grams/kg/day. Muscles aged sixty years or older require a higher dietary protein intake to stimulate muscle growth. Because of this, older people need to **both** stimulate muscle with resistance loads **and** increase their daily total protein consumption into the 1.2-1.4 gm/kg range. (Wolf 2006)

In 2013, the European Union Geriatric Medicine Society updated, evidence-based recommendations in the

PROT-AGE (Protein Needs With Aging) paper. PROT-AGE recommends seniors an average daily protein intake at least in the range of 1.0-1.2 g per kilogram of body weight per day (1.2 g/kg body weight/day). The expert panel further recommends both endurance and resistance-type exercises at individualized levels and higher protein intake (i.e., ≥ 1.2-1.5 g/kg body weight/day) for those who are exercising and otherwise active or have chronic illnesses. Those with kidney failure are an exception to this recommendation and may need to limit their protein intake. (Bauer 2013)

For those who have no dietary protein restrictions, set aside one day to check your protein intake. Take, for example, the following scenario. Jane might eat a bowl of shredded wheat, milk, orange juice and coffee for breakfast. Assuming Jane weighs 60 kg, or 132 lbs, how can we make sure that Jane consumes enough protein to stimulate muscle growth?

Convert from pounds to kg: **132** divide by 2.2 lbs/kg = 60 kg

Find daily protein needs: 60kg x **1.4** grams protein/day = **84 grams**

Breakfast example of protein:

1 cup of milk = 8 grams

1 serving of shredded wheat = 5 grams

Juice + coffee = 0 grams

8 + 5 = 13 grams!

Thirteen grams out of 84 grams per day is less than **16%** of her daily protein need! She must make up the rest over lunch, dinner and other snacks. A good number of people eat salad for lunch, but a garden salad with tomatoes, carrots, throw in even avocados doesn't even add up to one gram of protein! An egg is 6 grams. High protein Greek yogurt is 12 grams. Add either of those for lunch and you still haven't got even one-third way to the required daily protein to grow muscle. Those with lactose intolerance who avoid cheese or milk are another group potentially short on protein. One of the easiest solutions to ensure adequate dietary protein might be to buy a container of whey protein powder to supplement your exercise program.

Ensuring enough protein intake is especially paramount for thin prediabetics. Compared to obese prediabetics, thin diabetics are characteristically deficient in the muscle department, stemming from a proportionately larger contribution of muscle insulin resistance. For them, not eating enough protein might require the body's recycling of precious muscle protein to meet their exercise needs. Consequently, strenuous exercise paired with insufficient protein can potentially lead to loss of muscle mass! While a plethora of weight training websites and articles tout finer aspects of dietary protein, for seniors, as of 2017, the scientific studies aren't in agreement regarding *when* seniors should supplement with protein after strength training. More age-generalized studies suggest that protein intake with some carbohydrate should follow strenuous exercise within four hours, so consider timing your supplements accordingly!

Because skeletal muscle by lean body mass makes up 40-55% of the total weight of a typical healthy man, it is not hard to see why inactivity-related loss of skeletal muscle mass might lead to insulin resistance. Beginning after age 40, we lose 5% of muscle mass each decade. By the time we have reached the end of the seventh or eighth decade, the loss of muscle mass accelerates, leaving some 50% of our original muscle mass. The young, strong, 155-pound male has a peak muscle mass of roughly about 80 lbs. By contrast, an 80 year-old woman may have a mere 30 pounds muscle remaining. This eye-popping lifetime loss explains why half of women over the age of 65 who break a hip, are prone to falls and even after successful surgery, don't have the strength to walk again. Recall that muscle is the chief storehouse of glucose, and so it also explains why glucose levels tend to rise with age.

Who still needs to chase mastodons?

For our bodies to return to our healthy evolutionary heritage, we must restore the physique and physiology that our ancestors enjoyed. Most people are comfortable "exercising the heart," perhaps using an elliptical machine – an exertion possibly akin to chasing mastodons. Upon hopping off the elliptical, these poorly informed individuals might think that they are done exercising. Perhaps, they don't see the need for promoting other aspects of caveman muscles, since we no longer chuck spears nor heave large rocks. They are dead wrong. While clean water, vaccinations and modern medicine have vanquished vast swaths of infectious diseases, metabolic diseases have taken their place.

To counter emergent lifestyle diseases such as Type 2 diabetes, we require exercise, especially resistance. I invite you to think of exercise as prescriptive, not unlike medicine dispensed from a pharmacy. The best training programs have a scientific basis and a defined goal – not a semi-random collection of what could be called "Stupid Human Tricks." A well-rounded exercise program should include aerobic exercise, flexibility, agility and resistance training for all muscle groups. Resistance exercises include: body weight-based exercise such as yoga, resistance bands, free weights, and machines like a universal weight gym. For this section, we'll limit our discussion to movement related, or dynamic muscle exercises, and why they are the most well-established treatment of insulin resistance.

Unlike aerobic exercise, resistance training aims to damage muscle fibers, but only slightly and in a safe, controlled manner. Compared with aerobic exercise, resistance training needn't be lengthy, only difficult enough to make microscopic muscle tears. In contrast to aerobic exercise, the recovery period is more important as the resistance exercise itself. Sufficient recovery time permits the body to rebuild stronger and bigger muscle fibers. Often, older people recoil from the thought of lifting weights, having a mental image of backbreaking manual labor and possibly getting hurt. Consequently, allowing adequate recovery time is part of the plan. Unceasing and overwhelming workloads frequently disabled generations of manual laborers. Properly executed, resistance training is a repetitive cycle of controlled, microscopic muscle fiber injury followed by prescribed healing – this is the genius of resistance exercise science. There is a bonus for those with obesity. By way of incurring a need to rebuild, resistance exercise increases the body's protein and calorie requirements. So even in periods between exercise, the metabolism is in an anabolic construction phase -- a near continuous caloric energy consumption mode.

If you can now set aside the fear of injury, let's recall an earlier chapter praising the value of muscle fatigue. Muscle fatigue correlates with the drawing down of muscle glycogen and therefore is a super indicator for a training goal. Those in the kinesiology field term this "training to failure." It sounds a bit like "training to fail," but the theory makes sense, even though the words sound scary. It means that you should always try your best, without losing proper form or having to use other muscles or untoward movements. In practice, one might be able to lift the bar eight times, but by the ninth time, it only moves up a little. Assuming you are not holding your breath or doing anything else wrong, you can give yourself a pat on the back for a job well done. The inability of being able to budge the bar means the glycogen level has dropped below threshold levels. You have essentially flushed the enzyme system, clearing glucolipotoxins and banished insulin resistance for 48 hours.

When performed properly, both aerobic and resistance training cycle down glycogen stores, reversing the insulin resistance roadblock using two separate, yet complementary methods. The muscle cells change their indifference to glucose and begin to respond eagerly to the glucose flowing by in the bloodstream. This theory has been confirmed by the success of High Intensity Interval Training (HIIT) to treat prediabetes and diabetes. HIIT research studies have shown intense aerobic exertion for very short periods of time equals the effect of prolonged, less intense aerobic training. When either are added to a progressive resistance exercise-to-exhaustion regimen, increased number of glucose transport molecules (GLUT4) become available to reverse insulin resistance. No previously sedentary person or diabetic should start HIIT without first talking with a physician. By contrast, no one is too old or too infirm for resistance training according to the US Health and Human Services recommendations for exercise. In fact, with rare exceptions, (and I can't even think of one) every adult should be doing some form of resistance training.

This is the solution for the person who is in a phase of impaired metabolism, diabetes, prediabetes or Metabolic Syndrome. Resistance exercise when added to aerobic exercise and proper diet offers the promise of reversing insulin resistance. We seek to use resistance exercise to fix an abnormal glucose and lipid metabolism. Even though we'll share the gym with a younger crowd who primarily seek bulging muscles, if we follow through with our goals, our side benefit will be stronger, higher quality muscles that will allow us to live longer and independently.

Chapter 7: Enough Theory, Let's hear Practice

What kind of results can I expect from this exercise program?

A reasonable question to ask is, "How much can one expect to improve with exercise?", which is not the same question as, "How much will I improve with this medication, Doctor?" Medications have been shown to improve glucose control, and often by increasing the dosage of a medication may achieve a certain level of control. Even so, glucose control does not equate to halting disease progression. Diabetes is a progressive disease, despite and even with the best medications, a point often glossed over during patient counseling. Complications from diabetes are only somewhat prevented with the best medical care. On the other hand, exercise treats the underlying cause. Especially early in the insulin resistance continuum, there may be no limit to the improvement possible. It just takes patience and persistence.

Most exercise studies have monitored outcomes such as insulin resistance, GTT, fasting blood glucose or Hemoglobin A1C. Please recall, as a cascading process, improvements are reflected first in insulin resistance, then triglycerides, GTT, Hemoglobin A1C and fasting blood sugar is last measurable change. Keep in mind that fasting blood sugar measures liver insulin resistance, something not directly affected by muscle insulin resistance. The liver has an independent sensing and output of overnight glucose from muscle, so fasting blood sugar might not be changed by this regimen.

One study, DARE (*Diabetes Aerobic and Resistance Exercise*, Sigal 2007) kept track of changes of Hemoglobin A1C and medications after 22 weeks, which is a relatively short period of time to exercise. Hemoglobin A1C improved in the combined aerobic and resistance exercise group by a startlingly 0.9 percent. For reference, metformin is said to reduce Hemoglobin A1C by 1.1 percent. (Hirst 2012) In the DARE study, the number and dose of diabetic drugs were reduced for those exercisers compared to those not exercising. In contrast to medications, improvements with exercise continue to accrue over time. Continued exercise beyond 22 weeks should exceed the effect of metformin. Should I add, "Your own mileage may vary."?

For my generation of physicians focused on treating diabetics with drugs, meeting the original goal meant achieving almost normal glucose levels. As intuitive that sounds, not only is it a nearly impossible target, it also is a bad idea. Here's a point you might find interesting: no expert panel currently recommends even attempting to achieve a normal level of equal or <5.6%, which is considered normal or even an A1C of 5.7–6.4% (which is the prediabetes range).

Attempting to entirely normalize glucose with medication is fraught with pitfalls. The required effort is Herculean, and the risk of dangerous side effects such as hypoglycemia sometimes life-threatening. Consequently, 2013 ADA guidelines call for diabetic control to a Hemoglobin A1C level of 7% or less. Sometimes even higher target levels are appropriate for older folks (8%). Patients with longer projected lifespans should shoot for lower levels of A1C, less than or closer to 6.5% A1C. For reference, normal glycohemoglobin levels are less than 5.7%. At a certain point, diabetic medications become too large a factor in an increasingly brittle system that produces less homegrown insulin. High insulin resistance paired with a high dose of injected insulin is a less stable system, unless a continuous pump sensor system is used. Even if one is in a late stage diabetes, exercise can help diabetics become less brittle. Let's examine how.

Dr. Bacchi compared an hour of exercise in Type 2 diabetes patients with an implanted continuous glucose monitor. The dark line in the chart above, is the patient's nighttime glucose level without exercise and

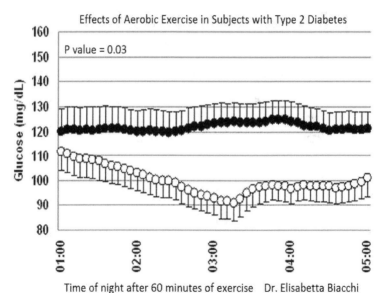

Effects of Aerobic Exercise in Subjects with Type 2 Diabetes

Time of night after 60 minutes of exercise   Dr. Elisabetta Biacchi

the white circles are the result of one hour of exercise the day before. These patients had been aerobically exercising about three months before test monitoring.

Two consecutive nights were compared after exercising during the evening prior. Glucose levels were lower throughout the night. Of course, in real life diabetics should be careful not to exercise immediately before going to bed. The take home message is that aerobic exercise can lower blood sugar dramatically for hours afterwards. By combining aerobic with resistance exercise, you can enjoy even longer lasting results. (Bacchi 2012)

Diabetes is not simply a "lack of enough insulin" disease. There are a host of other hormones at abnormal levels, including glucagon, and incretins to name a few. Trying to supplement every known metabolic defect in diabetes with a drug presumes complete knowledge and leaves open the real possibility of treating a surrogate marker – going back to our "surrogate marker" concern. Our goal is to return metabolism as close to normal as possible, not primarily to return it back to a lab test value, such as with glucose or triglycerides. All of the abnormalities of diabetes should revert toward normal if the underlying problem is addressed.

Exercising back to a normal metabolic state is quite doable for those early in the disease process but probably not for those in the later stage of diabetes because the weakened pancreas has much fewer Beta cells. Still studies show that exercise is the single best choice. For those with prediabetes or even early diabetes, a Hemoglobin A1C of less than 5.7% is achievable with the methods in the DARE study. (Sigal 2007) The earlier that one begins serious training, the more likely that insulin resistance will normalize.

Breaking the unending stress on overworked insulin secreting Beta cells can stave off or prevent their premature demise. Without breaking the stress on Beta cells, the few remaining Beta sells will be unable to sustain a normal system, even if insulin resistance is later reversed. So, it's better to get going earlier rather than later since patients have a better chance of normalizing their insulin resistance just by beginning serious training. In fact, if you are in the Metabolic Syndrome stage, the odds that training will improve your insulin resistance are 9:1 — this means that you will be 100% better off by exercising than you would be if you didn't. (Phillips 2014)

A little pain now or much more later

Exercise takes grit. Admittedly injury are potential side effects and count on sore muscles the next day. On balance however, exercise addresses the core issues, not medications. I encourage you to take the long view. It took a long time for you to get to this point. As long as you are making steady progress, every day in the right direction counts. Yo-yo dieting and fat farm style exercising has been shown to be without enduring gains and even metabolically detrimental. But most people are correct to start off with aerobic exercise.

For obese people with a BMI >32, focusing upon 150 to 300 minutes a week of aerobic exercise and diet might offer the best first steps. Simply angling into one of the universal weight resistance machines can be challenging, and not to mention, put one at risk of injury. Consider sitting resistance exercises such as a leg press machine if moving presents a challenge. Usually the muscles below the waistline are strong, and the ones above the belt can be exercised with mainly dumbbells or bands. Water aerobics or swimming are great ways to avoid getting hurt at this stage.

For those who are more easily mobile, the Fitbit has filled a niche for encouragement toward, taking the more steps toward exercise. Just the same, I would like for us to recognize that the Fitbit is no more than a computer which gives people an artificial but concrete incentive. Simply counting steps on a device is not enough in the long run as a comprehensive plan. Sometimes you need to enlist a comrade in arms – someone who shares your goal. Make a friendly contest or compact. Stay in touch with them, share progress notes by text, Facebook – whatever makes you comfortable. If you have successfully begun, then consider yourself on the way to getting to a better place, keep the momentum going and pointed up.

As far as motivation goes, fun is overrated. For myself and most physicians, going into the hospital or clinic isn't fun, but it definitely is rewarding. On a higher plane, rewarding trumps fun. Sometimes one has to do things which might not fall into the fun category. Brushing teeth regularly doesn't fall into the fun category, but part of good hygiene. Exercise may at first feel like taking a shower, washing clothes and brushing your hair. However, a funny thing often happens after a few weeks to months of daily exercise. Studies spanning over two decades have affirmed that people feel happier when regularly exercising. In fact, regular exercise has even been suggested as therapy for depression. (Craft 2004) Sometimes it takes a bootstrap motivation method to overcome inertia. Bootstrapping starts with an unfamiliar but easy commitment. One reason that home gyms often fail is that they are located at home. Don't worry about the whole process of exercise. Block out the hour and commit to getting to the gym. The act of driving to an exercise facility is easy enough. Once you are there, all you need to do is to get out of the car, go inside and try to fit in. One step puts you smack into the next step. Sometimes people get psyched out thinking about the big hill rather than mediating with a mantra of "just cranking the pedals around for another ten revolutions, 1, 2, 3, 4, 5, 6, 7, 8, 9, 10," followed by another ten . . . .

For those who are non-obese or have a BMI < 32, adding resistance training to aerobic exercise with more protein in your diet should be the next logical step. This brings me to a question from women at Q&A's, which at first surprised me, "Will I get bulky (muscles)?" To which I usually quip in my usual jesting fashion, "No, did you want them?" Bulking up is just about impossible by the time women hit your mid 40's without the combination of East German steroids or some unusual medical condition. Almost no amount of resistance exercise will cause you to be mistaken for Arnold, the former actor turned Governor of California. It just won't happen.

What will happen is that your clothes in the back of the closet will beckon as you will slim from the inside, starting with the central fat apron surrounding the omentum and intestines. The subcutaneous fat will thin, but not disappear. You can start moving those favorite clothes up toward the front of the closet for the upcoming season.

You just qualified for Prediabetes or Metabolic Syndrome, now what?

Presuming your doctor has and is checking your Hemoglobin A1C at least annually and found you to be in the range of 5.7–6.4%, several studies show that you can prevent further sliding. Traditional aerobic exercise and weight loss can prevent slightly less than half of the cases of prediabetes from becoming diabetes.

These studies have achieved this with diet, weight loss and 150 minutes per week of moderate aerobic activity. *You can do better than these odds.* One reason is that these statistics are from institutional studies. They have only limited numbers of exercise machines and they have to tailor the exercises for the study, not for the individual. As an individual, you can exercise to better effect than study participants.

Dozens of studies have shown the superiority of combined resistance and aerobic exercise programs over those relying only on diet and aerobic exercise. The traditional low-fat, low-calorie diet coupled with lower intensity activity such as walking works - to a limited degree. This traditional treatment approach may no longer be optimal because it does not include more recent findings from dietary and exercise research. If you have read this far, you already know why.

Additional words of caution for diabetic exercisers

Diabetic patients should exercise, but when the following conditions are present, first get medical clearances in particular:

1. Poorly controlled high blood pressure

2. Foot sores or prior injuries

3. Nerve damage or impaired feeling especially in the feet

4. Retinal complications (back of eye)

5. Other infections or illness when present

In 2015, the American College of Sports Medicine issued new preparticipation guidelines for exercise. (Riebe 2015) The panel worried the previous guidelines might have actually been a barrier to exercise. You can see the guidelines directly at this link:

http://journals.lww.com/acsm-msse/Abstract/2015/11000/Updating_ACSM_s_Recommendations_for_Exercise.28.aspx

In general, there are three considerations. The expert panel's new model for exercise preparticipation health screening focuses on three factors: current level of physical activity; the presence of signs or symptoms of known cardiovascular, metabolic, or renal disease; and the eventual desired exercise intensity. If you are already exercising without worrisome symptoms, but have hypertension, prediabetes or diabetes, then the guidelines suggest that no medical clearance is necessary for moderate intensity exercise. If the same person wishes to advance to high-intensity exercise, then medical evaluation is suggested. On the other hand, if you have been inactive and have hypertension, prediabetes or diabetes, then the guidelines suggest medical evaluation prior to starting light to moderate-intensity exercise. Please remember that if you have any worrisome signs or symptoms, or wish to engage in HIIT, then you should seek medical evaluation. While any exertion increases the risk of heart arrhythmia, there is an intelligent way of going about this.

When I was a teenager, before becoming a physician, my family went to see this soon-to-be retired doctor in Fairfax, Virginia. I think my father liked the guy because he usually prescribed antibiotics freely at my father's behest. In spite of this practitioner's seeming lack of control over his prescribing pad, the venerable doctor was an exercise fear-monger.

In his waiting room, the doctor delighted in posting various obituaries, news stories and medical articles about individuals suddenly expiring while exercising. It's true, James Fixx, the famous runner author of "The Complete Book of Running," died when running, although he was at one time, obese, smoked and had an enlarged heart. The risk for death during aerobic exercise is increased about six times over the same period of time sitting, and an exercise death occurs once every 1.5 million times during vigorous physical exertion in men, even more rarely in women.

But fear not. Cardiac rehab is another name for exercise prescribed for heart attack and heart failure patients. Exercise is appropriate for just about anyone, even those with known heart disease and it is best to be cautious rather than overenthusiastic. The risk of a heart attack is proportional to the degree of exertion, especially unaccustomed levels of exertion. Light-to-moderate intensity exercise is therefore less of concern. The take home message is that "easy does it" is safe.

Gradually increasing the intensity over time is the smart way to aerobic workout. The heart needs time to adapt to higher expectations. The short-term risk of exercise is more than offset by the long-term benefits.

Studies done on the lifetime return on exercise are astounding. If one were to start exercising at or above the national exercise guidelines in their 40's, a 7:1 return on lifespan investment is average. (Moore 2012) In other words, for every one minute of exercise, health statisticians have calculated you will live another seven minutes longer. Not seven minutes of time being watching life while sitting, but still able to bound up the steps of the Acropolis to gaze across the city of Athens. (There was no elevator service when I last visited.) That's enjoying a long health-span!

Finally, diabetics should have a snack on hand and perhaps a glucometer in the event of feeling lightheaded from hypoglycemia. With exercise, many patients will notice an immediate improvement in their glucose levels and will need tapering of their medications. High-intensity exercises in particular cause a prolonged and delayed decrease in glucose. Exercise mimics a shot of insulin to the extent that exercising too late in the evening can result in hypoglycemia while sleeping, a potentially dangerous situation.

Inspect your feet, toes and toenails daily for blisters, redness, ingrown nails and signs of infection. Many diabetics regularly see podiatrists because they have lost some feeling in their feet. It takes only a minute when changing into some good exercise shoes to make sure nothing is amiss with the two front feet!

Like anyone who exercises, drink water frequently to keep ahead of thirst. Thirst is a late, not an early sign of a state of low hydration. US Army physiologists recommend drinking at regular intervals as opposed to drinking whenever thirst suggests. (Montain 2010)

Difference between physical exercise and physical activity – "A goal without a plan is simply a wish."

On more than one occasion, someone has asked me, "I garden, doesn't that count as physical activity?" Admittedly, some activity is better than no activity. Gardening is better than planting yourself in front of a television or computer. Nonetheless, studies have shown that women who regularly garden retain only grip strength, losing muscle strength elsewhere and bone density. (Reynolds 1999) The same goes for housework, a British study found it to be woefully inadequate to maintain muscle mass, (Murphy 2013)

If you wish to achieve something, you need more than desire. You need to be smart about it, making sure it has some scientific basis and that it makes sense for you. It must be attainable and relevant to you. If you know you can't stick with the program, then choose another program. It should have some kind of metric of progress, something measurable – otherwise, how do you know you are making progress?

Look at those older than you. How did those with a planned regimen fare compared with those with general activity? Physical activity and physical exercise both involve movement. Sometimes physical activity requires us exert ourselves, move faster, or strike a tennis ball with a racquet held in one hand.

Consider a professional tennis player. Roger Federer's right forearm muscles have been compared to a baseball bat and his left to a tire iron. This is the outcome of a repetitive physical activity which focuses only on one motion. The same can be said for cycling, running or cross country skiing. None of us would aspire outside of playing professional level tennis to train only one and not both arms.

Activities should also be evaluated from a safety aspect. Tennis involves twisting, sudden dashes and stops. This is a recipe for injury after age 40, as any weekend softball player will tell you. Sprains commonly arise from unexpected forces exceeding the limits of tendons. A good physical exercise is a measured challenge to our muscles, nerves, bones and tendons. The exercise should encourage adaptations of greater speed, resiliency and flexibility. When all four structures muscles, nerves, bones and tendons, advance in lock-step, we rarely get injured. In fact, this kind of gradually progressive exercise prevents us from getting injured. In other words, exercise should be a planned activity.

I would go further and say, ***"Physical exercise is a planned activity intended to induce physiologic and cell level adaptations."*** Those body adaptations are a response to the increased stepped challenges and the goal of exercise. The goal might include any combination of strength, endurance, balance, improved metabolism, decreasing high blood pressure, increasing the speed of reflexes, relaxation or fending off dementia. To be effective, exercise needs to be designed with a goal in mind. A physical activity won't reliably get you where you might want to go.

Adaptation: A force your body understands

Adaptation has been a recurrent key concept throughout this book. The purpose of exercise is to demonstrate to your muscles their present inadequacy, in other words, give muscles enough of a stimulus to drive change. Change can come from challenging muscle from various aspects. Kinesiology and exercise experts have summarized into an acronym FITT: Frequency, Intensity, Type and Time. Exercisers can vary the type of exercise they perform as well as how frequently, how intensely, and for how long the adaptive change of exercise can take place. Restated, one might exercise longer, harder or use a different method. Although this is easier said than done, High-intensity Interval Training (HIIT) is a huge time saver. Those who have exercised for a while and enjoy challenges probably will do well with High-intensity Interval Training. One resistance example might be a triceps exercise performed with dumbbells versus with a cable machine. When strength plateaus, trainers often switch training modalities (types) in order to leapfrog temporary stasis.

Most people misinterpret the 150 minutes as a target exercise guideline. Many who are trying to lose weight will require up to 300 minutes a week of exercise to make meaningful inroads. For those who do not have the luxury of five hours, accumulating the time in ten-minute intervals is a great strategy. Ten minutes has been shown to be approximately the minimum amount of time for exercise to have a physiological aerobic effect. Sitting should likewise be limited.

Taking exercise breaks throughout the day is an excellent way to refresh the mind and body. The American Diabetes Association has a new recommendation for 2016: get up from sitting every 30 minutes. The thinking behind this is glucose management is improved by breaking up periods of sitting. Active muscles like to be fed. For planned activities, writing a time and date, or day of the week can help mentally commit to a regimen.

To achieve your goal, physical exercise has a crafted and designed structure. Take for example someone who bicycles. A common question that I get is, "I bicycle, does that count as exercise?" If your goal is to be able to lift your carry-on luggage into the overhead bin, then the obvious answer is "No."

What if your goal is to maintain cardiovascular fitness? Then the answer is "Depends." An average bicycle can easily go 10 miles per hour, about the top safe speed for riding in any suburban green way or shared pedestrian path. To achieve that speed on level ground, for most people requires an exertion of about 40-50 watts or about 3-4 METS. (MET: Metabolic Equivalent of Task. Roughly, 1 MET was originally conceived as the same energy burn rate of quietly sitting. That is still close enough for our discussion.) To give you a comparison, normal walking at 3 mph is about 3 METS and jumping rope is 10 METS. This kind of urban bike riding is relatively light when compared with recognized, established aerobic exercise recommendations. Moderate-intensity exercise begins at about six METS.

You might have seen this funny bumper sticker which shouts to a tailgater, "If you can read this, you're too close!" I would like the sign in the cartoon below taped

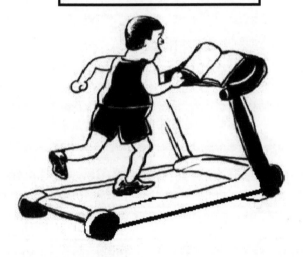

If you can read that book, you aren't going fast enough!

to treadmills, "If you can read your book, you're not exercising hard enough!" If you are in the gym, try to get the most out of your invested time by taking it up a notch. Exercise is all about adaptation. Remember that hills are your friend? If one has a plan to ride up a 3% grade, half mile-long hill at 10 mph, that is a worthy goal. This SMART goal has a specific, measurable, achievable, rewarding and time-based outcome. Part of a plan to gradually increase the grade, distance or speed, (150 watts or ~10-11 METS) makes it more akin to metabolically useful and meaningfully intense exercise plan. By raising the bar, setting a progressive goal of riding steeper for longer, we're showing the proverbial carrot to our muscles and increasing strength and stamina. We're not talking about an inspirational goal, but incrementally achievable goal. "The next bigger hill is your next best friend," is shorthand for this kind of progressive aerobic training.

A counter yet familiar example of "lowering the bar" are Snow Birds with two homes. Perhaps you know of Snow Birds, who upon returning from wintering in Florida find their New York home's stairs a challenge? That's the result of only a few months' worth of deconditioning.

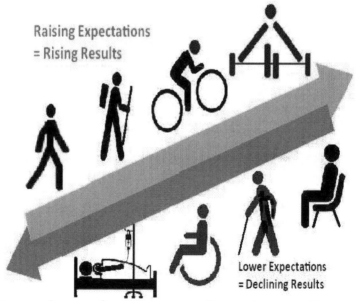

"Demand more from your muscles, get more. Demand less, anticipate . . . ."

Quite a few scientific studies have tested the best set of exercises for achieving metabolic results. The more useful studies detail the method of how the goals were achieved. The most reliable studies have had their results reconfirmed and have compared the results with control groups. With this in mind, the last part of this book has synthesized the best studies into a model program.

The best time to plant a tree is 20 years ago. The second best time is now.

You should have a clear idea of your goal when starting an exercise program. If your goal is to improve glucose and fat metabolism, then you should concentrate on large muscles. All muscles increase proportionately with the same amount of effort. Exercising large muscles has a greater effect on improving metabolism than the same effort applied to small muscles.

The largest muscle groups in the body are chest, shoulders, back, abdomen and legs. These axial muscles are located along the vertical axis of your body from your chest (core) down to your calves. In this way, our metabolically focused regimen differs from the muscle builder who might focus on the chest, abs and showman biceps.

Resistance exercise challenges your muscles to adapt to lift progressively heavier loads more times. Preventing muscles from "resting on their laurels" at any level is central to steady improvement. The easiest way to do this is to keep track with either paper and pencil or some software like the Jefit app for the computer or smartphone. (I use the electronic formats because it keeps track of exercise volume and calculates intensity.) Record keeping demonstrates a conscientious attitude toward constant improvement.

Learning how to breathe properly is especially important to a diabetic who might have eye problems. Improper breathing can raise blood pressure for everyone, but is especially damaging for diabetics with retinopathy, a type of eye problem. In general, holding one's breath is not the best idea, as it tends to raise blood pressure more than otherwise. A good way to remember is to blow out as if you are trying to blow the weight up during the repetition.

While you may not be able to perform some exercises, you should not consider yourself exempt from exercise. The latest US Health and Human Services guidance of 2008 says:

> *"Adults with disabilities, who are able to, should also do muscle-strengthening activities of moderate or high-intensity that involve all major muscle groups on 2 or more days a week, as these activities provide additional health benefits."*

If you have specific limitations, work around them. Seek the guidance of a physical therapist, kinesiologist or well-informed trainer. Don't be left out.

At the risk of repetition, a recap of metformin. This drug has been found to mimic exercise in several ways. Researchers from the University of Alberta found that those patients who were taking metformin and exercising seem to cancel each out. While research is ongoing, reversing insulin resistance with exercise does not seem to help those taking metformin as much.

Some researchers have found that metformin puts a cap on exercise performance. Patients taking metformin tend to reach the same heart rate or exercise intensity at lower workloads. There is evidence that metformin blunts benefits of exercise at improving insulin sensitivity and inflammation. Stay tuned and don't change medications without consulting your healthcare provider.

General Exercise Guidelines – Be selfish, invest in yourself

The major health organizations have coalesced around a central core of aerobic and resistance recommendations. Most people are only familiar with the aerobic recommendation:

"Adults should do at least 150 minutes (2 hours and 30 minutes) a week of moderate-intensity, or 75 minutes (1 hour and 15 minutes) a week of vigorous-intensity aerobic physical activity, or an equivalent combination of moderate- and vigorous intensity aerobic activity. Aerobic activity should be performed in episodes of at least 10 minutes"

The five day, 30-minute (5 x 30 = 150 minute) recommendation is for the average healthy adult to maintain health and reduce the risk for chronic disease. For weight loss, more time (300 minutes) or more intensity may be necessary. Aerobic exercise is a great way to warm up muscles first before the next phase, resistance exercise. Here is the second part of the recommendations:

"Adults should also do muscle-strengthening activities that are moderate or high-intensity and involve all major muscle groups on 2 or more days a week."

While the eventual strength training goal should not be for light intensity, one should start out gently to become accustom to the exercise, learn to do it correctly and then gradually build strength. Lifting is an exercise in mindfulness; you are instructing your body how to lift something heavy. Likewise, three sessions is better than two sessions a week. Furthermore to build the most strength, each session should focus on a muscle group not emphasized in the previous session. That's what we personally recommend. In this way, more recovery time is allowed following a more muscle stimulating workout.

Some DIY'ers do the same routine every time. Not only is that boring, but rotating among the various muscle groups allow them to rest. If there is some overlap, your regimen should exercise the same muscle groups in different ways. Believe it or not, the same muscles are made up of small bundles of fibers with slightly different orientations, which improve when pulling in new directions. A Prisoner Squat challenges slightly different muscles than a Goblet Squat.

For older people, 48 hours should be the minimum rest interval between exercising the same muscle groups. Muscle get stronger when recovering from the stimulus which is strength training. Since it takes longer to recover than in the past, we recommend you give your body longer time between re-challenging the same muscles compared with exercise routines for younger people. The recovery and rebuilding period cannot be overemphasized. The most commonly injured joint during resistance training is the shoulder. Studies report that exercises such as the "overhead press" and the "dumbbell chest fly" are particular culprits setting back older folks. Ligament tears happen when trying to handle too much resistance, too soon. Easy does it. Shoulder impingement syndrome commonly occurs when tendons rub in narrow spaces and become inflamed. Older bones tend to grow bone spurs, so think range of motion exercises. Add in weak muscles showing up as rounded, drooping shoulders and you can understand why often shoulders need care. Physical therapists often prescribe shoulder girdle strengthening exercises as a result. Please advance shoulder exercises gingerly if this might apply to you.

As a general guideline, large muscles should be exercised before small muscles and multiple joints should be exercised before single joints. For example, squats should be performed before leg extensions. A squat exercises hips, knees and ankles – three joints. Although it is less widely accepted, some researchers believe that exercising large muscles release myokine substances into the bloodstream which help all muscles grow faster than if this order were reversed.

Muscles, bones and tendons along with soft tissue fascia which envelope muscle, replace themselves over time. Rebuilding time cycles for these body parts are in this ascending order: Muscles, bones, followed last by tendons and soft tissue fascia. Muscle cells react fastest to exercise. Bone takes a longer time and tendons take longest. Too often, someone starts exercising, gets stronger and tears a ligament or the fascia, which is the soft tissue sleeve surrounding a muscle. The injury puts an immediate stop to workouts and undoes recent progress. Moral of the story: *It takes a longer time to strengthen ligaments and soft tissue, give them time to catch up with faster growing muscle.*

Commonly the day after resistance training soreness will be noted upon awakening. Delayed Onset Muscle Soreness (DOMS) is thought to be the result of microscopic tears in the muscle cells. These tears cause mild swelling, some pain, inflammation, and perhaps stiffness, perhaps lasting between to 48 to 72 hours. While joint pain signals a need to back off or back down, muscle pain is generally okay. Muscles will be the sorest after the first few training sessions, but, over time, DOMS occurs to a decreasing degree as resistance training progresses. And, in fact, some find that pretreating DOMS with protein supplements helps reduce the soreness. Therefore, another reason to start training with lower intensities is to lessen the severity of DOMS.

Start with weights well below your ability and learn proper form from a trusted trainer. Studies have shown **exercise volume** matters most when it comes to growing muscle:

Exercise volume = total weight lifted

= number of repetitions x number of sets x pounds of weight

You can lift half the weight twice as many times and have the same exercise volume. So studies have shown the same muscle bulk results when up to six sets are performed. Lifting lighter weights for more sets can almost achieve the same results. Intensity should be your focus, do your best and lift until you no longer can budge the weight. I usually lighten the load and repeat the process on the last set until the final weight is 50% of my peak load.

Tendons are a different story. Patellar tendon strength can't be improved simply by walking faster – ligaments need to experience more stress. Too many middle age people tear ligaments (sprain joints) doing previously trivial tasks. Strength training all joints prevents decaying tendons, an added bonus. Strengthening studies done on tendon show impressive gains approaching 60% improvement, but only with higher weight loads. Dr. Grosset's research showed higher loads, more than 40% and probably in the 70-80% of 1-RM range were required to stimulate tendon strengthening. (Grosset 2014) Now is a good point to introduce the measurement of load in resistance training.

A useful measure of strength is 1-RM, or "One Rep Maximum" – the theoretical maximum weight that you can lift once. It doesn't come from lifting a dangerous amount of weight once, but from counting the number of times one can lift a lighter weight. As one gets stronger, the 1-RM goes higher. 1-RM can be calculated from a chart:

% of 1RM	Number of repetitions
100	1
95	2
90	3
85	5
80	8
75	10
70	12
65	15

As in the example for tendon strengthening, you would aim to lift some poundage up to eight times. If you can perform eight reps but no more than eight reps, then it is according to the chart, at the 80% of 1-RM difficulty. But if you can perform 60 lbs for eight repetitions *and only eight*, then 1-RM is calculated from the chart as 60/0.80 = 75lbs. For comparison, 40% of 1-RM corresponds to being able to perform 50 reps, definitely not a burdensome heavy load. To improve tendon strength for example, one needs to lift somewhere between 50-80% 1-RM range.

You should start out with low weights and a larger number of repetitions. After about some period of adaptation, you should think about increasing the weight. I recommend staying within an 8-15 repetition range. (65% to 80% 1-RM range) Target eventually being able to perform two or three sets, but starting out with a single set. The eventual goal is to keep the workout short but always challenging. In other words, you should be performing repetitions until you can't anymore. I like to successively drop the weight down at this point and keep trying. This has the effect of recruiting the most muscle units and burning down the glycogen.

Just as we might measure aerobic intensity with an age-adjusted heart rate or Borg scale of Perceived Exertion, (see Glossary under "Exercise Intensity") the percentage of 1-RM is a measure of resistance exercise load. Progressive resistance training hopes to achieve continuous quality improvement, similar to the Japanese approach to car manufacturing called, "kaizen."

Suppose you have been performing two sets of eight repetitions of "Lat pull downs" at 60 lbs for several weeks. Early on, the two sets were challenging, but thanks to your persistence, the last set is now easy. In our example above for a theoretical one-time lift, you could lift (1-RM), 75 lbs, as calculated for this effort. How to increase to the next level?

Variation #1: You could try to increase the number of repetitions per set to nine repetitions. This is a stamina – strength compromise. This is my personal recommendation. I try to stay within an 8-15 repetition range. Over time, I gradually increase the number of repetitions to 15 per set. After 15, I might drop down to 8, but at a higher weight and increase the number of repetitions. You could get fancy and simultaneously drop down the number of repetitions and increase the weight. You want to raise the 1-RM equivalent slightly higher (<5% increase).

Variation #2: You could try to increase the number of sets to three. In the third set, it may not be possible to perform eight repetitions, but any number you can perform with good form is progress. Your goal in this case is to increase stamina.

1-RM sounds a bit unwieldy, but smart phone apps such as Jefit automatically do the calculations. With progressive resistance training, it is a given that the 1-RM will rise. It is a good feeling to see the change.

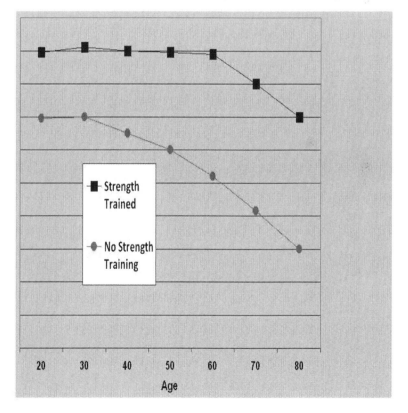

80 can almost be as strong as 30

A sad, yet commonly held wrongheaded view is, "We're all going downhill and nothing is going to change that." While in the long run we're all going to die, over the short run, we can make regular gains. Dr. Darren Candow and his group from the University of Regina in Canada, weight trained a group of 60-71 year old men for 22 weeks. Afterwards, the group was indistinguishable in strength from a group of untrained young men. (Candow 2011) This type of study has been repeated elsewhere with 75-year-old men and women, with similar strength gains. (Stewart 2014) Say you are older than that? The study has been repeated with 76 to 92-year-olds! (Yarasheski 1999) While Father Time steadily taxes our hypothetical, optimal body, we can almost always be stronger and more capable than if we did nothing.

If it's important, you'll find a way. If not, you'll find an excuse.

If you have picked up this book, and read this far, you have demonstrated commitment in reversing or preventing a decline in your health. You understand the purpose of strength training. Having a goal is requisite and having a plan is the next important thing to have. Oftentimes physicians say, exercise more, or move around more. (I suppose that is what the Fitbit has accomplished.) Physicians, myself included have been remiss in providing a concrete road map to follow – which is the very reason this book exists.

Some of us, in fact very few of us have the self-discipline to take on the exercises in this book and follow through to achieve what is truly possible. Knowing yourself and how well (or not!) you have done in the past is a good guide.

There are lots of "tricks" for following through. These might include using a cell phone or computer program, putting money down for a gym membership or enlisting an exercise buddy for spiritual support. If it is a gym membership, surprisingly, the distance to the gym usually determines long-term success; pick one that is close. Most important is getting into a routine and sticking with it. Sometimes joining a national chain where you can exercise even while traveling will keep you on track when on the road. Consider a bonding "couple's time together" if your significant other is in the same boat. (They'll either pull you up or drag you down typically.) Make a pact with a like-minded pair of friends and double team this exercise goal. For many of you, in fact, the great majority, it will also take a trainer to help you take the plan and make it a life-changing experience.

Consider this analogy to financial planning. Many people recognize the value and need for long-term retirement planning. They don't wish to spend time educating themselves about investing or tax planning and willingly pay someone thousands of dollars a year to take care of it. Your health is worth more than money. But are you willing to invest the willpower to keep yourself on track? If that financial planner or tax accountant was well worth your money, then maybe a trainer might be too.

Trainers, like financial planners, provide value – only unlike financial planners, the kind of investment that they provide you with could be life-changing. Resistance training requires a self-conscious mindset, one which can be difficult to master at least initially without an outside observer. Contrasted with aerobic exercise, where people might try to get lost in the reverie akin to a runner's high, weight training takes concentration and attention to proper initial and final positions, overall form, timing of movement, and proper breathing in order to set a solid foundation for subsequent improvements. It is actually not a simple task to keep all these in mind, even when performing movements in front of a mirror.

Trainers also are famous for their skill in encouragement. They know how to gently get you to try your level best. They ensure we have gained the most out of our workout by "giving it our all." Many people under-train by not challenging themselves consistently or sufficiently. Lower intensities often fall short of effecting those wonderful changes. Exercise each resistance set to exhaustion, but before you lose good form.

Exercising with trainers, obviously costs more than doing it yourself. That could be viewed as a positive. After plunking down money, we are "dollar bound" to finish out the sessions. The trick is to gain enough knowledge and habit of training for it to become part of our lifestyles. Some can cut back working on with a trainer after gaining enough knowledge and discipline. Sometimes that initial investment in ourselves is the kick-start that we need.

One of the most important reasons to work with a trainer is injury prevention. Too often I have encountered an enthusiastic, silver-haired athlete start a program, overdo it and be set back by injury. Of course, I don't have to tell you it takes longer to bounce back. Not only can a trainer keep you from straining ligaments, they can help you work around injuries that crop up. Say you sprained your wrist, a trainer can keep you on track by exercising the other parts until recovered.

All this said, I should add important disclaimers. Learning good form and selecting the right starting weight and number of repetitions are difficult to do on your own. While mirrors allow oneself to watch for proper form, sometimes the viewing angles aren't perfect and learning incorrect form from the outset leads to problems down the road. Consequently, even an experienced trainer will ask another trainer to check their form when trying out a new exercise. Form is paramount because you are intuitively teaching your body how to manage the simultaneous handling of weight with movement. When your body has intuited this knowledge, you are much less likely to injure yourself picking up something or falling.

If you have known heart disease, limit the intensity of aerobic exercise initially and increase in slow increments. Cardiac Rehab monitors and helps establish what might be a safe threshold. Since anyone might have undiagnosed coronary artery blockage, exertional or resting arrhythmia's, valve or heart muscle or lung or even joint issues, always check with your health provider before increasing or embarking on a new program.

If you are unaccustomed to exercise, then gradual

increases, "easy does it" is the watch phrase. You want to change the trajectory of your life, but it is unlikely that your body will immediately adapt to the full sessions below. The duration, intensity and number of all exercises below are general and eventual target guidelines, which the average person with no known restrictions can attain. We strongly advise that you take this program to a trainer, maybe a physical therapist if you have physical limitations, or a qualified healthcare professional if you have cardiac concerns to see if these exercises are suitable for you.

Exercises have a well-established naming system. If you are the DIY type, many excellent videos can be found on YouTube, where you can type in the name of any exercise on the site's search bar and see variations. Finally, good luck. I hope you will have a copy of lab reports, new clothes or astonishment from your doctor to brag about.

Chapter 8: The FIRST Exercise Program©

This scientifically-based, model exercise **7 day, Comprehensive Regimen** was created in conjunction with Dylan Reilly, an Exercise Physiologist MS, CPT and Cory Malone, MA, CPT. They own and operate Isles Fitness (http://islesfitness.com) in Punta Gorda, Florida. We have two regimens which are similar. The **Resistance Only Regimen** is a single table grid with A,B,C days is designed for those with access to a commercial gym such as LA Fitness, Planet Fitness or Gold's Gym. The C Day can be performed at home if desired.

Both training regimens have distilled exercise protocols from multiple successful, published medical studies. The 7 day Comprehensive Regimen is organized by the order of exercise days, rather than days of the week. It is designed so you can exercise every day without straining any body part. I strongly recommend you literally make a habit of exercising every day. In this way, skip days become the exception. When acclimated, the regimen should take between 45-60 minutes or less per day.

The program has exercises, which can be done at home, as well as those that might require more specialized equipment. The exercise protocol is a structured example of a complete routine designed to target metabolic deficiencies and can be tailored to all fitness levels. No fitness program, including the program outlined is appropriate for all individuals. Therefore, it is recommended to seek the advice of a fitness professional before implementing any exercise regimen. They can substitute a more appropriate exercise which could exercise the same muscle group.

Some notes:

1. The pages may not print out well, or be easy to copy. Here is a pair of links, which lead to the same spot on the internet where you can print out a copy of the exercises, as they should appear: http://bit.ly/2rPROIO https://www.dropbox.com/sh/x4lb6z0zkiex2q0/AAC 5Q7or_oO8YkyOM3Wa0rjRa?dl=0

2. Prior to each session perform 5-10 min of full body aerobic exercise warm-up (elliptical, rower, air dyne bike of low/moderate intensity) and 5 min of total body active stretching.

3. Ideally, start with 2 sets of 10-15 reps. When you can easily perform 3 sets of 15-18 reps for each exercise to exhaustion, advance the weight by the smallest increment or add another set.

4. Attempt to limit rest time between sets to no more than 30 seconds

5. Each weight session is to be followed by 5 minutes of aerobic exercise (elliptical, rower, treadmill at preferably moderate/high intensity) and 5 min of total body static stretching

6. Supersets are paired exercises, such as Triceps & Biceps, Hamstring & Knee extensors.

7. Supersets are done as alternating pairs. Example: Leg followed by Core, then again Leg followed by Core would be two Supersets.

8. Don't forget aerobic exercise intensity matters. Set your eventual goal to eventually maintain a Borg RPE intensity of 13 and for 1-2 minute short bursts, reach a Borg RPE intensity of 14 or more where you can only recite the *Pledge of Allegiance* a few words at a time. (feel free to choose your own mantra!) If you use a heart monitor, personalize your heart rate thresholds using this method.

9. Increase your water consumption especially on Days 4 and 7

Resistance Only Regimen					
Exercise	Muscles	Day	Set (s)	Reps	Weight
Low back extension	Low back	A			
Bird Dog	Core	A			
Seated Row	Upper back	A			
Shoulder Shrug	Shoulder	A			
Knee Extension	Leg	A			
Hamstring Curl	Leg	A			
Supine Bench Press	Chest	A			

Leg Press	Leg	A			
Lat Pulldown	Upper back	B			
Barbell Deadlift	Multijoint	B			
Sitting Bench Press	Chest	B			
High Front Lift/Row	Shoulders	B			
Bicep Curls	Arms	B			
Triceps Kickback	Arms	B			
Torso Rotation	Low back	B			
Squats	Multijoint	C			
Lunges	Multijoint	C			
Abdominal	Abdominal	C			

Crunches					
Plank	Core	C			
Superman	Core	C			
Scissor Kick	Abdominal	C			

	Facility Training Day 1 of 7	Date			
	• Warm up Aerobic exercise	5-10 mins			
	• Total Body Active Stretching	5 mins	Set (s)	R e p s	Weight
	Push- Flat Bench Dumbbell Chest Presses				
	Pull- Bent Over Rows (barbell or dumbbells)				
Superset	*Leg- Squats (dumbbells or barbell)				
	*Core- Low Plank (30-60 sec)				
	Push- Triceps Push Downs				
	Pull- Dumbbell Biceps Curls				

Superset	*Leg- Dumbbell Step Ups				
	*Core- Superman				
	• Moderate/High Intensity Cardio	5 mins			
	• Total Body Static Stretching	5 mins			

	Home Training Day 2 of 7 5-10 min of low/moderate intensity full body cardio warm-up and 5 min of total body active stretching	Date	Sets	Reps
Active Stretching Warm Up 20 sec for each	Arm Circles			
	Trunk Twists			
	Alternating Cross Body Toe Touches			
	Pulsing Squats			
	Stretch Bends (squat into calf raises)			
	Standing Alt Elbow to Knee Crunch			
Lightweight Dumbbell	Front Shoulder Raises			
	Alternating One Arm Rows			
	Sumo Deadlift High Pulls			

	Alternating Biceps Hammer Curls			
	Triceps Kick Backs			
Abs (on ground) 2 rounds 30 sec each	Straight Leg Toe Touches			
	Side Lying Hip Abduction			
	Air Bike (with alternating elbow to opposite knee crunch)			
	Hip Thrusters (ground)			
Cardio for 20 minutes	Walking, Biking, Swimming Moderate to High intensity (hard to carry on a conversation)			
	• **Static stretching for 5-10 min with 15-20 sec holds**			

	Facility Training Day 3	Date			
	• Warm up Cardio	5-10 mins			
	• Total Body Active Stretching	5 mins	Set (s)	R e p s	Weight
	Push- Dumbbell Military Presses				
	Pull- Lat Pull Downs				
Superset	*Leg- Alternating Dumbbell Lunges				
	*Core- Physio Ball Straight Crunches				
	Push- Bench Dips				
	Pull- Dumbbell Lateral Shoulder Raises				

Superset	*Leg- Hamstring Curls				
	*Core- Back Extensions				
	• Moderate/High Intensity Cardio	5 mins			
	• Total Body Static Stretching	5 mins			

Days 4 and 7: (Facility or at Home)

Cardio: Moderate Intensity 20-30 min

Active Stretching

Arm Circles: With arms straight and to sides, make small slow arm circles with palms out. Gradually increase size of circle, then reverse direction – approximately 20 seconds in each direction.

Twist and reach: to each side, outstretch left arm and reach while rotating horizontally across body to the right, reverse position continuously, 30 seconds total.

Floor to Sky – stand in slightly squat stance with straightened legs, but not locked out knees, reach and touch floor (feel stretch in hamstring) and then reach forward and upward with both hands toward the sky (feel stretch in trapezius, the upper shoulder muscles on either side of the neck) repeat 10 times, 2 – 3 seconds pause in each direction.

Perform 15 body weight squats, 10 squat bends (squat and then lift heels as you stand up to be on your tip toes), and 5 light squat jumps (land softly, jump no more than 2 inches off floor).

Butt Kicks – shifting from foot to foot, kick your own butt with each heel (stretching the quad) – about 20 – 30 seconds total.

Static Stretching:

Seated V Stretch– Sit with legs straight and V spread. Reach up towards ceiling so you feel a stretch in upper back. While stretching upper back, bring arms forward and reach towards feet, keeping posture (stretching through back) and bringing chest as far forward while reaching towards feet. Hold for 20 – 30 seconds. Staying down move hands to your right leg (right hand outside, left hand inside). Try to compress your chest to your thigh – repeat on left side

Butterfly Stretch – sit in butterfly upright as much as possible, pressing thighs down to the floor while pulling in your feet , facing insole to insole. Keep back upright as possible.

Shift to Dead Frog – while lying on back, arms extended overhead, keep bottom of feet pressed together. Bring knees together and relax (like butterfly) and then slowly push feet away from lower body (while keeping feet together). Hold position for 10 – 15 seconds, and push the feet further away – continue until you cannot keep feet touching

Figure Four Stretch – While laying flat, bend left knee - with left foot flat on floor. Take right leg and cross it over the top of the left thigh. From this positions take your right hand, reach it between your legs and wrap it around the front of left knee. Reach left hand around and lock fingers with right hand. Pull back and hold for 30 seconds. Repeat for other side

Quad Stretch- Lay on right side and grasp left forefoot with left hand, pull heel towards your butt – keeping knees and hips in alignment for 10 seconds. Relax for 5 seconds and repeat 5 times. Repeat on left side.

	Facility Training Day 5 of 7	Date			
	• Warm up Cardio	5-10 min			
	• Total Body Active Stretching	5 min	Sets	R e p s	Weight
	Push- Dumbbell Chest Flies				
	Pull- Dumbbell Reverse Flies				
Superset	*Leg- Barbell Straight Leg Dead Lifts				
	*Core- Lying Leg Raises				
	Push- Push Ups (incline if necessary)				
	Pull- Pull Ups or Inverted Rows				

Superset	*Leg- Dumbbell or Kettlebell Swings				
	*Core- Bird Dogs				
	• Moderate/High Intensity Cardio	5 mins			
	• Total Body Static Stretching	5 mins			

	Home Training Day 6 of 7 5-10 min of low/moderate intensity full body cardio warm-up and 5 min of total body active stretching	Date	Sets	Reps
Active Stretching Warm Up 20 sec for each	Arm Circles			
	Trunk Twists			
	Alternating Cross Body Toe Touches			
	Pulsing Squats			
	Stretch Bends (squat into calf raises)			
	Standing Alt Elbow to Knee Crunch			
Lightweight Dumbbell Exercises 2 rounds of 12	Front Shoulder Raises			
	Alternating One Arm Rows			
	Sumo Deadlift High Pulls			
	Alternating Biceps Hammer Curls			
	Triceps Kick Backs			
Abs (on ground)	Straight Leg Toe Touches			
	Side Lying Hip Abduction			

ea ch	Air Bike (with alternating elbow to opposite knee crunch)			
	Hip Thrusters (ground)			
Cardio for 20 minutes	Walking, Biking, Swimming Moderate to High intensity (hard to carry on a conversation)			
	• **Static Stretching 5-10 min with 15-20 sec holds**			

Glossary:

1-RM: A sports science concept, this is defined as a predicted one-repetition maximum of weighted resistance. In practice, it is considered unsafe to lift this much weight. This is used this to establish a resistance exercise intensity, expressed as a percentage of 1-RM.

Aerobic exercise: Also known as Cardio exercise, a sustained exercise, as jogging, swimming, or cycling, that aims to strengthen the heart and lungs, by improving the body's utilization of oxygen, i.e. heart and lung function.

Anabolic resistance: The diminished muscle building response to ingestion of protein. Although it comes with aging, it can be induced with immobilization in young people such as in the case of casts.

Anaerobic exercise: The highest intensity of exercise achieved in resistance training to exhaustion, when no more repetitions can be done. In aerobic exercise, it is an unsustainable exercise rate when at some point, one needs to "catch my breath."

Anabolism: The metabolic chemical reactions where simpler substances are combined to form more complex molecules. Anabolic reactions usually require energy.

Anabolic state: A condition that is usually associated with the net building up of protein or in our discussion, muscle.

Atherosclerosis: The blockage of blood vessels. It begins as a collection of fat laden inflammatory cells in the inner layers of the blood vessel. Over time, it becomes larger and eventually calcified. When it occurs in the blood vessels of the heart, it is called "Coronary Artery Disease".

Carbohydrate: One of three macronutrients, required in large quantities. (others are protein and fat) This is the larger group composed of simple sugars, starches and less well digestible fiber.

Cardiovascular: The heart and blood vessels of the body. Usually blood vessels are classified into arteries and veins.

Cardiovascular diseases: Atherosclerosis, coronary heart disease, heart muscle, valve, rhythm disorders, high blood pressure, lipid disorders.

Cholesterol Panel: (aka Lipid panel) A standard blood test composed of total cholesterol, triglyceride, HDL (High-Density Lipoprotein) and LDL (Low Density Lipoprotein). LDL can be measured directly or is calculated from the other components.

Coronary Artery Disease: Atherosclerotic blockage or narrowing of the heart artery, may cause symptoms of angina. When the blockage suddenly narrows, a heart attack and usually a sudden heart rhythm disturbance, or arrhythmia occurs.

Catabolism: The metabolic chemical reactions that result in the breakdown complex organic molecules into simpler substances. Compare with Anabolism.

Catabolic state: A condition that is usually associated with net loss of proteins. Common examples are weight associated dieting or lack of adequate nutrition, especially protein.

Creatine phosphate: Also known as Phosphocreatine is a compound that serves as a lightening quick, reserve of high-energy in skeletal muscle and the brain.

DASH diet: A diet plan emphasizing fruits and vegetables, low-fat and nonfat dairy products, nuts, beans, and adding in more protein and/or heart healthy fats.

Deconditioning: The physiological change resulting from inactivity, prolonged bed rest or a sedentary lifestyle.

Endurance exercise: A type of aerobic exercise where sub maximal muscle contractions are designed to improve aerobic capacity.

Exercise: A structured physical program intended to induce specific physiologic and morphologic adaptations. This is to be distinguished from physical activity.

Exercise intensity: Generally percentage of maximum heart rate is used as the most common gauge of aerobic exercise intensity, simply because it is simple. A better gauge is the Borg Rating of Perceived Exertion which is on a scale from 6 to 20. 6-9 is barely considered exercise, like strolling slowly at leisure ("la, la, la"), light (10-13) can carry on a lively conversation, moderate (14-16) means that I can speak only in short phrases, and intensity 17-20 can't be sustained indefinitely, a high or anaerobic stage.

Fatty acids: This is a general term for a subtype of circulating fats, the most commonly recognized type triglyceride.

First Law of Thermodynamics: Law of Conservation of Energy, states that energy cannot be created or destroyed in an isolated system.

Glucotoxicity: The theory that high levels of glucose are toxic and damaging to cells of organs. Combination of high levels of fat and glucose is known as glucolipotoxicity.

GLUT-4: This is a glucose transporter molecule. It is manufactured in packets in the cells and integrates into the cell surface membrane. GLUT-4 is thought to the be principal structure affecting insulin sensitivity in muscle. There are other types of glucose transporter molecules which are in other organs.

Glycogen: The starchy substance stored in muscle, liver and other tissues as the main storehouse of carbohydrates. When called upon, it breaks apart to form glucose.

Hemoglobin A1C: This is a test which averages the glucose level over about three months. In recent years, certain manufacturers of this test have received FDA approval for use as a diagnostic test for diabetes in addition to the previous use as a monitoring test for diabetes. In certain types of people, such as those with abnormal hemoglobin, sickle cell, the test interpretation is a little less straightforward.

High Intensity Interval Training, (HIIT): a form of exercising training strategy alternating short periods of intense anaerobic exercise with less-intense recovery periods

Incretins: a class of signaling hormones secreted by the intestinal tract which influence glucose and fat metabolism.

Isometric exercise: a type of strength training in which the joint angle and muscle length do not change during contraction. Usually compared with dynamic/isotonic exercises.

Kinesiology: The scientific study of human body movement. Kinesiology focuses upon physiological and biomechanical mechanisms such as the physics of movement, orthopedics; strength conditioning; such as physical and occupational rehabilitation therapy. This should distinguished from applied kinesiology which some regard as quackery.

Lipid: Another name for fat.

Lipotoxicity: The theory that high levels of fat are toxic and damaging to cells of organs. Some include glucose at high levels as toxic, glucolipotoxicity.

MET: Metabolic Equivalent of Task. Originally, 1 MET was considered as the same energy burn rate quietly sitting, now it is slightly different. For our purposes, it is close enough. It allows us to generalize about the amount of effort for every person. Two METS means twice the burn rate as sitting on a couch watching TV. If you ever had a heart treadmill test, they usual measure the intensity in METS which are controlled by the steepness of the incline and speed of the belt.

Pathophysiology: My specialty! The study of how normal physiology becomes soured. In other words, the mechanism by which disease come about and cause problems.

Physiology: The study of the normal functioning of the body from the cells on up to how organs interact with each other. Exercise physiology is the study of how the body changes with exercise.

Progressive exercise: The program of exercises aims to increase physical strength, through the lifting of progressively heavier weight or resistance or metabolic efficiency through stepped increases in aerobic exercise intensity.

Resistance exercise: A broad form of exercise requiring one to exert force against a resistance. Generally it is nearly synonymous with Strength training but in our case, we are seeking an improved metabolism as a goal, versus an outward performance change in muscle.

Resting Metabolic Rate: This is a theoretical measurement of baseline metabolic rate if no activity were taking place. In practice, this usually is not a normal test condition, following rest and a 12 hour fast. A major flaw in this concept is it assumes no ongoing protein repair, such as muscle following resistance training is taking place or more mitochondria are being added from aerobic exercise.

Sarcopenia: The state of having generalized less of skeletal muscle mass and strength. It has been associated with deconditioning, physical inactivity, poor quality of life and increased risk for death.

Strength training: The use of resistance methods with the goal of improving physical muscle performance. Commonly employs free weights, resistance bands, body weight or machines.

Superset: Two exercises paired together, performed successively without rest. According to theory, this creates more metabolic stress, and increased energy expenditure in a shorter period of time. Common pairings include chest and back, quads and hamstrings, and biceps and triceps.

Triglycerides: The main component of the biochemical class known as fatty acids, a type of fat found in blood and tissue. The body uses it for energy and storage.

Additional Reading:

Sex Differences In Whole Body Skeletal Muscle Mass
Measured By Magnetic Resonance Imaging And Its
Distribution In Young Japanese Adults
Abe T, Kearns CF, Fukunaga T
Br J Sports Med 2003;37:436–440

Glycemic index in chronic disease: a review
Augustin LS
European Journal of Clinical Nutrition (2002) 56, 1049–
1071

Insulin Resistance Predicts Mortality in Non-Diabetic
Persons in the United States.
Ausk KJ, Karlee J. Ausk, MD
Diabetes Care June 2010 vol. 33 no. 6 1179-1185

Differences in the Acute Effects of Aerobic and
Resistance Exercise in Subjects with Type 2 Diabetes:
Results from the RAED2 Randomized Trial.
Bacchi E, Negri C, Trombetta M, Zanolin ME, Lanza M,
Bonora E, et al.
PLoS ONE (2012) 7(12): e49937.
doi:10.1371/journal.pone.0049937

A New Method for Non-Invasive Estimation of Human
Muscle Fiber Type Composition
Baguet A, Everaert I, Hespel P, Petrovic M, Achten E,
Derave W
PLoS ONE (2011) 6(7): e21956.
doi.org/10.1371/journal.pone.0021956

Comparison of Aerobic Versus Resistance Exercise Training Effects on Metabolic Syndrome (from the Studies of a Targeted Risk Reduction Intervention Through Defined Exercise - STRRIDE-AT/RT)
Bateman LA, Slentz CA, et al.
Am J Cardiol 2011;108:838 – 844

Evidence-Based Recommendations for Optimal Dietary Protein Intake in Older
People: A Position Paper From the PROT-AGE Study Group
Bauer J
JAMDA 14 (2013) 542e559

Is lost lean mass from intentional weight loss recovered during weight regain in postmenopausal women?
Beavers KM, Lyles MF, Davis CC, Wang X, Beavers DP, Nicklas BJ
Am J Clin Nutr 2011;94:767–74

Cardiometabolic Risk After Weight Loss and Subsequent Weight Regain in Overweight and Obese Postmenopausal Women
Beavers DP, Beavers KM, Lyles MF, Nicklas BJ
Gerontol A Biol Sci Med Sci. 2013 June;68(6):691–698

Exercise training-induced triglyceride lowering negatively correlates with DHEA levels in men with type 2 diabetes.
Boudou P, de Kerviler E, Erlich D, Vexiau P, Gautier JF.
Int J Obes Relat Metab Disord. 2001 Aug;25(8):1108-12.

Metformin and exercise in type 2 diabetes: examining treatment modality interactions.
Boulé NG, et al.
Diabetes Care. 2011 Jul;34(7):1469-74
.

Does metformin modify the effect on glycaemic control of aerobic exercise, resistance exercise or both?
Boulé NG
Diabetologia. 2013 Nov;56(11):2378-82.

Novel and Reversible Mechanisms of Smoking-Induced Insulin Resistance in Humans
Bergman BC, et al.
Diabetes; Dec 2012; 61, pg. 3156-66

Accurate assessment of beta-cell function: The hyperbolic correction
Bergman R, Ader M, Huecking K, Van Citters G
Diabetes; Feb 2002; 51, pg. S212

Short-Term Heavy Resistance Training Eliminates Age-Related Deficits In Muscle Mass And Strength In Healthy Older Males
Candow DG, Chilibeck PD, Abeysekara S, Zello GA
Journal of Strength & Conditioning Research: Feb 2011 – Vol 25:2 p 326-333

A Randomized Controlled Trial Of Resistance Exercise Training To Improve Glycemic Control In Older Adults With Type 2 Diabetes
Castaneda C, Layne F
Diabetes Care 25: 2335-2341, 2002

Mechanisms for greater insulin-stimulated glucose uptake in normal and
insulin-resistant skeletal muscle after acute exercise
Cartee GD
Am J Physiol Endocrinol Metab 309: E949–E959, 2015

Statin-Induced Muscle Damage And Atrogin-1 Induction Is The Result Of A Geranylgeranylation Defect
Cao Peirang, et al.
FASEB J. 23, 2844–2854 (2009)

Effects of Aerobic and Resistance Training on Hemoglobin A1c Levels in Patients
With Type 2 Diabetes: A Randomized Controlled Trial
Church Timothy S. , et al.
JAMA. 2010;304(20):2253-2262

Altered Myokine Secretion is an Intrinsic Property of Skeletal Muscle in Type 2 Diabetes
Ciaraldi TP
PloS ONE 11(7)

Skeletal muscle lipid deposition and insulin resistance: effect of dietary fatty acids and exercise
Corcoran MP, Lamon-Fava S, and Fielding RA
Am J Clin Nutr 2007;85:662–77.

Comparison of Serum Lipid Values in Subjects With and Without the Metabolic Syndrome
Cordero A
Am J Cardiol 2008;102:424–428

The Benefits of Exercise for the Clinically Depressed
Craft LL
J Clin Psychiatry 2004;6:104-111

Effects of Exercise Modality on Insulin Resistance and
Functional Limitation in Older Adults: A Randomized
Controlled Trial
Davidson Lance E, et al.
Arch Intern Med. 2009;169(2):122-131

Insulin Resistance, Lipotoxicity, Type 2 Diabetes And
Atherosclerosis: The Missing Links. The Claude
Bernard Lecture 2009
DeFronzo RA
Diabetologia (2010) 53:1270–1287

Effects of Weight Loss by Diet Alone or Combined
With Aerobic Exercise on Body
Composition in Older Obese Men
Dengel DR
Metabolism Vol 43, No 7 (July), 1994: p 867-871

Pathogenesis and pathophysiology of accelerated
atherosclerosis in the diabetic heart
D'Souza A
Mol Cell Biochem (2009) 331:89–116

Effects of Ramipril and Rosiglitazone on Cardiovascular and Renal Outcomes in People With Impaired Glucose Tolerance or Impaired Fasting Glucose: Results of the Diabetes REduction Assessment with ramipril and rosiglitazone Medication (DREAM) trial
The DREAM Trial Investigator
Diabetes Care 31:5 (May 2008): 1007-14.

Age-related anabolic resistance after endurance-type exercise in healthy humans
Durham William J., et al.
FASEB J. 24, 4117– 4127 (2010).

Aerobic and Strength Training in Concomitant Metabolic Syndrome and Type 2 Diabetes
Earnest Conrad P.
Med Sci Sports Exerc. 2014 July; 46(7): 1293–1301

Vegetarianism, female gender and increasing age, but not CNDP1 genotype, are associated with reduced muscle carnosine levels in humans
Everaert, I; Mooyaart, A; Baguet
Amino Acids April 2011 , Volume 40, Issue 4, pp 1221–1229

Exercise and nutritional interventions for improving aging muscle health
Forbes SC, Little JP, Candow DG
Endocrine (2012) 42:29–38

The Influence Of Resistance Training On Patients With Metabolic Syndrome —

Significance Of Changes In Muscle Fiber Size And Muscle Fiber Distribution
Geisler S, Brinkmann C, Schiffer T, Kreutz T, Bloch W, Brixius K
Journal of Strength and Conditioning Research 2011, 25(9)/2598–2604

Immobilization induces anabolic resistance in human myofibrillar protein synthesis with low and high dose amino acid infusion
Glover Elisa I, et al.
J Physiol 586.24 (2008) pp 6049–6061 6049

Diagnosis and Management of the Metabolic Syndrome: An American Heart Association/National Heart, Lung, and Blood Institute Scientific Statement 2005 ATPIII Revised Criteria
Grundy SM, et al.
Circulation 112, 2735–2752

Influence of exercise intensity on training-induced tendon mechanical properties changes in older individuals
Grosset JF
AGE (2014) 36:1433–1442

Insulin-Resistant Prediabetic Subjects Have More Atherogenic Risk Factors Than Insulin-Sensitive Prediabetic Subjects
Haffner SM, Mykkänen L, Festa A, Burke JP, Stern MP
Circulation. 2000 Mar 7;101(9):975-80.

Increasing Exercise Intensity Reduces Heterogeneity of
Glucose Uptake in Human Skeletal Muscles
Heinonen I, Nesterov SV, Kemppainen J
PLOS One 2012 Dec 20,
https://doi.org/10.1371/journal.pone.0052191

The Muscle-Specific Ubiquitin Ligase Atrogin-1/Mafbx
Mediates Statin-Induced Muscle Toxicity
Hanai Jun-ichi , et al.
The Journal of Clinical Investigation Volume 117
Number 12 December 2007

What causes the insulin resistance underlying obesity?
Hardy OT
Curr Opin Endocrinol Diabetes Obes. 2012 April ; 19(2):
81–87.

Exercise as a therapeutic intervention for the
prevention and treatment of insulin resistance
Hawley JA
Diabetes Metab Res Rev 2004; 20: 383–393.

Exercise training-induced improvements in insulin
action
Hawley JA, Lessard SJ
Acta Physiol 2008, 192, 127–135

Skeletal Muscle Composition and Its Relation to
Exercise Intolerance in Older Patients With Heart
Failure and Preserved Ejection Fraction
Haykowsky MJ, Kouba EJ, Brubaker PH, Nicklas BJ,
Eggebeen J, Kitzman DW
Am J Cardiol 2014;113:1211e1216

Quantifying the Effect of Metformin Treatment and
Dose on Glycemic Control
Hirst JA, Farmer AJ, Ali R
Diabetes Care, 02/2012, Volume 35, Issue 2

Insulin Sensitivity and Atherosclerosis
Howard G
Diabetes, 1988; 37:1595-1607

In Search of the Ideal Resistance Training Program to
Improve Glycemic Control and its Indication for
Patients with Type 2 Diabetes Mellitus: A Systematic
Review and Meta-Analysis
Ishiguro Hajime, et al.
Sports Med (2016) 46:67–77

The Role of Skeletal Muscle Glycogen Breakdown For
Regulation Of Insulin Sensitivity By Exercise
Jensen J, Rustad PI, Kolnes AJ and Lai YC
Frontiers in Physiology December 2011, Volume2,
Article112

Usefulness of the Triglyceride–High-Density
Lipoprotein Versus the Cholesterol–High-Density
Lipoprotein Ratio for Predicting Insulin Resistance and
Cardiometabolic Risk (from the Framingham Offspring
Cohort)
Kannel WB
Am J Cardiol 2008;101:497–501

Sugar Industry and Coronary Heart Disease Research
A Historical Analysis of Internal Industry Documents

Kearns CE, Schmidt LA, Glantz SA
JAMA Intern Med. 2016;176(11):1680-1685.
Skeletal Muscle Triglyceride
An aspect of regional adiposity and insulin resistance
Kelley DE, Goodpaster BH
Diabetes Care 24:933–941, 2001

Reduction In The Incidence Of Type 2 Diabetes With
Lifestyle Intervention Or metformin
Knowler WC
N Engl J Med, Vol. 346, No. 6 Feb 7, 2002

Glycogen Availability And Skeletal Muscle
Adaptations With Endurance And Resistance Exercise
Pim Knuiman, Maria T. E. Hopman, Marco Mensink
Knuiman et al. Nutrition & Metabolism (2015) 12:59

A single session of resistance exercise enhances insulin
sensitivity for at least 24 h in healthy men
Koopman R
Eur J Appl Physiol (2005) 94: 180–187

Does the Amount of Fat Mass Predict Age-Related Loss
of Lean Mass, Muscle Strength, and Muscle Quality in
Older Adults?
Koster Annemarie , et al.
J Gerontol A Biol Sci Med Sci. 2011 August;66A(8):888–
895

Appendicular Skeletal Muscle Mass and Insulin
Resistance in an Elderly Korean Population: The
Korean Social Life, Health and Aging Project-Health
Examination Cohort

Lee SW, Youm Y, Lee WJ, Choi W, Chu SH, Park YR, Kim HC
Diabetes Metab J 2015;39:37-45

Associations of Sarcopenia and Sarcopenic Obesity With Metabolic Syndrome Considering Both Muscle Mass and Muscle Strength
Jihye Lee, Yeon-pyo Hong, Hyun Ju Shin, Weonyoung Lee
J Prev Med Public Health 2016;49:35-44

Low-volume high-intensity interval training reduces hyperglycemia and
increases muscle mitochondrial capacity in patients with type 2 diabetes
Little JP
J Appl Physiol 111: 1554–1560, 2011

Disposition Index, Glucose Effectiveness, and Conversion to Type 2 Diabetes
The Insulin Resistance Atherosclerosis Study (IRAS)
Lorenzo
Diabetes Care (2010) 33:2098-2103

Sarcopenic Obesity Is Closely Associated With Metabolic Syndrome
Lu CW, et al.
Obesity Research & Clinical Practice (2013) 7, e301 – e307

The effects of increasing exercise intensity on muscle fuel utilisation in humans
Luc J. C. van Loon, et al.

Journal of Physiology (2001), 536.1, pp.295–304

Insulin Resistance Is an Important Risk Factor for
Cognitive Impairment in Elderly Patients with Primary
Hypertension
Ma Lina
Yonsei Med J 56(1):89-94, 2015

Current understanding of increased insulin sensitivity
after exercise – emerging candidates
Maarbjerg SJ
Acta Physiol 2011, 202, 323-335

Effects of CoQ10 supplementation on plasma
lipoprotein lipid, CoQ10 and liver and muscle enzyme
levels in hypercholesterolemic patients treated with
atorvastatin: A randomized double-blind study
Mabuchi H, Nohara A, Kobayashi J, Kawashiri M,
Katsuda S, Inazu A, Koizumi J
Atherosclerosis 195 (2007) e182–e189

Autoantibodies Against 3-Hydroxy-3-Methylglutaryl-
Coenzyme A Reductase in Patients With Statin-
Associated Autoimmune Myopathy
Mammen AL
Arthritis & Rheumatism Vol. 63, No. 3, March 2011, pp
713–721

Statin-Associated Autoimmune Myopathy
Mammen AL
N Engl J Med 2016;374:664-9

New insights into insulin action and resistance in the vasculature
Manrique C
Ann. N.Y. Acad. Sci. 1311 (2014) 138–150

Maximal Power Across the Lifespan
Martin JC, Farrar RP, Wagner BM, Spirduso WW
Journal of Gerontology 2000, Vol. 55A, No. 6, M311–M316

Live Strong And Prosper: The Importance Of Skeletal Muscle Strength For Healthy Ageing
McLeod M, Breen L, Hamilton DL, Philp A
Biogerontology DOI 10.1007/s10522-015-9631-7

Effect of Supervised Progressive Resistance-Exercise Training Protocol on Insulin Sensitivity, Glycemia, Lipids, and Body Composition in Asian Indians With Type 2 Diabetes
Misra Anoop
Diabetes Care, Volume 31, Number 7, July 2008 p1282

Effect of Supervised Progressive Resistance-Exercise Training Protocol on Insulin Sensitivity, Glycemia, Lipids, and Body Composition in Asian Indians With Type 2 Diabetes
Misra Anoop, et al.
Diabetes Care 31:1282–1287, 2008

Leisure Time Physical Activity of Moderate to Vigorous Intensity and Mortality: A Large Pooled Cohort Analysis

Moore SC, et al
PLoS Med 9(11): 2012 e1001335.
doi:10.1371/journal.pmed.1001335

Does doing housework keep you healthy?
Murphy MH, Donnelly PF, Breslin G, Nevill AM
BMC Public Health 13(1):966

Regulation of endogenous fat and carbohydrate
metabolism in relation to exercise intensity and
duration
Romijn, J. Coyle, L. S. Sidossis, A
American J Physiology 265(3 Pt 1):E380-91 · October
1993

Exercise-induced myokines and their role in chronic
diseases
Pedersen BK
Brain Behav. Immun. 2011, 25, 811–816

Crosstalk Between Exercise And Galanin System
Alleviates Insulin Resistance
Penghua Fang, Biao He, Mingyi Shi, Yan Zhu, Ping
Bob, Zhenwen Zhang
Neuroscience and Biobehavioral Reviews 59 (2015)
141–146

A Brief Review of Critical Processes in Exercise-
Induced Muscular Hypertrophy
Phillips SM
Sports Med (2014) 44 (Suppl 1):S71–S77

Hyperinsulinemia Predicts Coronary Heart Disease
Risk in Healthy Middle-aged Men
The 22-Year Follow-up Results of the Helsinki
Policemen Study
Pyorala M
Circulation. 1998;98:398-404

The Green Gym: An Evaluation of a Pilot Project in
Sonning Common, Oxfordshire Reynolds, Veronica,
Oxford Brookes University, 1999, Research Report No.
8, ISBN: 1 902606 05 1

Statin use in prediabetic patients: rationale and results
to date
Anastazia K, Evangelos C, Moses Elisa
Ther Adv Chronic Dis. 2015 Sep; 6(5): 246–251.

Insulin Sensitivity, Insulinemia, and Coronary Artery
Disease
The Insulin Resistance Atherosclerosis Study
Rewers M
Diabetes Care, Volume 27, Number 3, March 2004 p781

Updating ACSM's Recommendations for Exercise
Preparticipation Health Screening
Riebe D
Medicine & Science in Sports & Exercise, 2015 p2473

Type 2 diabetes in migrant south Asians: mechanisms,
mitigation, and management
Sattar N
Lancet Vol 3 December 2015, p1004

Effects of Aerobic Training, Resistance Training, or Both on Glycemic Control in Type 2 Diabetes, A Randomized Trial
Sigal RJ, et al.
Ann Intern Med. 2007;147:357-369

Review: diet interventions, with or without exercise, promote weight loss more than advice
Sharma AM
Evid. Based Med. 2008;13;41

Exercise, Abdominal Obesity, Skeletal Muscle, and Metabolic Risk: Evidence for a Dose Response
Slentz CA, Houmard JA, Kraus WE
Obesity (Silver Spring). 2009 December ; 17(0 3): S27–S33. doi:10.1038/oby.2009.385

Effects Of Different Modes Of Exercise Training On Glucose Control And Risk Factors For Complications In Type 2 Diabetic Patients. A Meta-Analysis
Snowling N, Hopkins W
Diabetes Care 29: 2518-2527, 2006

Mass Spectrometry-Based Proteomic Analysis Of Middle-Aged Vs. Aged Vastus Lateralis Reveals Increased Levels Of Carbonic Anhydrase Isoform 3 In Senescent Human Skeletal Muscle
Staunton L, Zweyer M, Swandulla D, Ohlendieck K
International Journal Of Molecular Medicine 30: 723-733, 2012

Responsiveness Of Muscle Size And Strength To Physical Training In Very Elderly People: A Systematic Review
Stewart VH, Saunders DH, Greig CA
Scand J Med Sci Sports 2014: 24: e1–e10

A Brief Structured Education Programme Enhances Self-Care Practices And Improves Glycaemic Control In Malaysians With Poorly Controlled Diabetes
Tan MY, Magarey JM, Chee SS, Lee LF and Tan MH
Health Education Research Vol.26 no.5 2011, 896–907

Prevention of Type 2 Diabetes Mellitus by Changes in Lifestyle among Subjects with Impaired Glucose Tolerance
Tuomilehto J, et al. The Finnish Diabetes Prevention Study Group
N Engl J Med 2001; 344:1343-135

The Underappreciated Role Of Muscle In Health And Disease
Wolfe, RR
Am J Clin Nutr 2006;84:475–82.

Skeletal Muscle Hypertrophy Following Resistance Training Is Accompanied by a Fiber Type – Specific Increase in Satellite Cell Content in Elderly Men
Verdijk LB, et al.
J Gerontol A Biol Sci Med Sci.
2009. Vol. 64A, No. 3, 332–339

Both resistance- and endurance-type exercise reduce the prevalence of hyperglycaemia in individuals with impaired glucose tolerance and in insulin-treated and non-insulin-treated type 2 diabetic patients
Van Dijk JW, et al.
Diabetologia (2012) 55:1273–1282

Muscle Mass, Muscle Strength, and Muscle Fat Infiltration as Predictors of Incident Mobility Limitations in Well-Functioning Older Persons
Visser M
Journal of Gerontology 2005, Vol. 60A, No. 3, 324–333

Developing A New Treatment Paradigm For Disease Prevention And Healthy Aging
R Winett, B Davy, E Marinik, J Savla, S Winett, S Phillips, L Lutes
TBM 2014;4:117–123 doi: 10.1007/s13142-013-0225-0

Effects of Diet and Exercise in Preventing NIDDM in People With Impaired Glucose Tolerance
The Da Qing IGT and Diabetes Study
Xiao-Ren
Diabetes Care; Apr 1997; 20, 4; p 537

Resistance exercise training increases mixed muscle protein synthesis rate in frail women and men 76 yr old
Yarasheski KE., et al.
Am. J. Physiol. 277 (Endocrinol. Metab. 40): E118–E125, 1999.

About the Author

William Shang, M.D. is a board certified physician with certifications from the American Board of Pathology and American College of Sports Medicine. He is presently directs two clinical laboratories at Cornell University and Ithaca College's Hammond Health Center Laboratory. A graduate of RPI-Albany Medical College's Combined Six Year Accelerated Program, he has over the course of his career been a USAF flight surgeon, primary care physician, hospital pathologist and coroner's physician for three New York counties. He initially trained in internal medicine at the USAF Wilford Hall Medical Center. After years of primary care, he completed training in anatomic and clinical pathology at George Washington University in Washington, D.C. The author can be contacted for speaking engagements or comments at:
wshang@yahoo.com

Acknowledgments

Writing a book can only be accomplished with help from others. I have been fortunate to have the book's biochemistry verified by two family friends, who are PhD level biochemists. Nathan Lindberg who teaches English writing at Cornell University took the initiative to guide me in reorganizing an early manuscript and guiding the text to professional and lay-language editing by Andrea Mendoza.

Speaking of patience, my wife Nora has heard an unceasing stream of trial explanations and analogies. The reader has been spared many a bad joke as a result. Finally my mother, who has been my cheerleader throughout. I think everyone should have a mom who thinks their kids have a unique gift to contribute to the world.